Overcoming the Pain of Inflammatory Arthritis

The Pain-Free Promise of Pantothenic Acid

Phyllis Eisenstein
Samuel M. Scheiner, Ph.D.

AVERY PUBLISHING GROUP
Garden City Park • New York

The advice in this book is based on the experiences of, and the pool of information available to the authors. It is not intended as a substitute for consultation with your physician or other health care provider. Because each person and situation is unique, the author and the publisher urge the reader to check with a qualified health professional when there is any question regarding appropriateness of any treatment.

The publisher does not advocate the use of any particular procedure, but believes that the information in this book should be available to the public.

Because there is always some risk involved, the publisher and author are not responsible for any adverse effects or consequences resulting from the use of any of the suggestions, preparations, or procedures discussed in this book. Please do not use the book if you are unwilling to assume the risk. For personalized advice, please consult a physician or other qualified health professional. It is a sign of wisdom, not cowardice, to seek a second or third opinion.

Cover design: William Gonzalez
Typesetter: William Gonzalez
In-house editor: Karen Hay

Avery Publishing Group, Inc.
120 Old Broadway
Garden City Park, NY 11040
1-800-548-5757

ISBN: 0-89529-902-X

Printed in the United States of America

10 9 8 7 6 5 4 3 2

Contents

To Alex, who told me this book should be written,
and to Judy, who helped to get it going.

ACKNOWLEDGMENTS

Writing a book like this requires help from a multitude of unanticipated sources. Many friends gave practical advice, answered questions in great detail by phone, or letter, or electronic mail, and even performed library research in some unexpected places. A number of total strangers were also generous with their time and efforts. This book could not have been written without them. To all of them, I give my thanks.

To James Huttner, M.D., for a long late-night conversation on pharmacology and for indispensable reference books.

To Barry Gehm, Ph.D., for explanations of scientific terminology and tireless searches of computer databases.

To Lev Yampolsky, Ph.D., for tracking down information on pantothenic acid research in the former Soviet Union.

To Dr. Andrej Moiseenok of the Biochemical Institute at Grodno, Belarus, for sending even more information on pantothenic acid research in the former Soviet Union.

To Rick Ralston of the Ruth Lilly Medical Library at the University of Indiana, for carrying Dr. Moiseenok's materials all the way home from Belarus and sending them on to me, and for digging up some articles I couldn't find in my local medical school library.

To Marina Ionina of the Chemistry Department of the University of Michigan in Flint, for her translation work.

To Donald R. Davis, Ph.D., of the Clayton Foundation Biochemical Institute at the University of Texas at Austin, for information on the work of Roger J. Williams.

To Avedon Carol, for trekking all over London, including the British Library, in search of books.

To Gail J. Jones of the Royal Society of Chemistry and Julie Beckwith of the Royal College of Physicians, for providing information on two of the British pantothenic acid researchers.

To Alice McMurtrie of the *British Journal of General Practice,* for providing an original article not available at my local medical school library.

To Alison Yates of the Food and Nutrition Board of the National Academy of Sciences, for sending me copies of various Food and Drug Administration publications.

To all of the volunteers who took part in our research study and all of those friends, relatives of friends, and friends of friends who have tried pantothenic acid on my word alone, for their curiosity and their trust.

And to my editor, Rudy Shur, whose interest and enthusiasm never failed to support my own commitment to this project.

PREFACE

Nearly forty million Americans have arthritis. They rely on a wide array of over-the-counter and prescription medications, from aspirin to naproxen sodium, from corticosteroids to gold compounds. But the great drawback of all of these drugs is that they have side effects that range from stomach upset to ulcers to liver damage and worse.

Arthritis sufferers are looking for something that will help them without hurting them. That's the reason for all the arthritis exercise and diet books we see at the bookstores. Proper exercise can moderate the pain, says one book. Finding the foods you're allergic to and eliminating them can get rid of your arthritis, says another. But exercise can be tough to stick with when you're in pain; and trying to determine your allergies—if they exist—can be a complicated, time-consuming, and frustrating experience.

I have arthritis. Long ago, I took phenylbutazone for it, a drug so dangerous that I had to have a blood test every week while taking it, to make sure my red blood cells weren't being destroyed. (Nowadays, it is no longer even listed in the standard book on prescription drugs, the *Physicians' Desk Reference*.) Now I take something else, something that allows me to walk, run, exercise, carry groceries, and vacuum my rugs without pain. That something else is not a painkiller and not an over-the-counter anti-inflammatory and not a prescription drug. It is a vitamin, available without a prescription, called pantothenic acid. For some years now, I have been on a quiet crusade on its behalf, urging fellow arthritis sufferers to give it a try.

Patricia, a librarian at a nearby university, recently sent me this electronic mail:

> Subject: Pantothenic acid.
>
> Phyllis, I have to share this one with you—I owe you more every year! I went dancing the other day—haven't been able to do that for quite some time. NO pain in the knees. I've always loved dancing and used to be quite good. Thanks for helping me to get something I love back in my life.

Like all the other people I've introduced to pantothenic acid, Patricia had never heard of it before I told her about it. There have certainly been no books about it, no articles in popular magazines devoted to it. It is one of the most obscure of the vitamins. Yet for me and for Patricia and for others, it has made an enormous difference in the quality of our lives.

A few years ago, my husband suggested I move away from the quiet crusade and write a book about this vitamin, so that more people would know to try it. I thought about that for a while. I am a writer; in the past, I had written novels, short stories, and book reviews, but never a nonfiction book. This was something important, though. Finally, I told him I would write the book, but only if I could find some real scientific research that supported pantothenic acid as an effective treatment for arthritis.

I found that research, and the book became a reality. My friend and collaborator, Sam Scheiner, became interested in the project while I was still preparing to write the book by reading mounds of scientific journals in a local medical school library. Together, he and I conducted our own research study on pantothenic acid and arthritis, which you'll read about in Chapter Seven. The Appendix is his—an explanation of that study for a reader who isn't accustomed to reading scientific journals. He also made many valuable suggestions for the rest of the book. But the bulk of the book is mine, and whenever you see the word "I," you'll know it's me, Phyllis, speaking from my own experience.

This is a book written by someone with arthritis for other people with arthritis. In it, you'll read my personal arthritis story, and then you and I will explore the disease itself, its symptoms and long-term effects, and the treatments generally used for it. Then we'll look at pantothenic acid and find out what it is, what it does in our bodies, and why a daily supply of it is vital to our health. We'll find out what foods are high in pantothenic acid and why depending on a balanced diet to give us enough of it is nearly impossible. We'll explore the scientific research that links pantothenic acid to the alleviation of arthritis pain, and we'll also look at the stories of real people who have tried it and consider it their own personal miracle. And then you'll come along with Dr. Scheiner and me as we conduct our own research study, and you'll see how our scientific results tallied with all of the other evidence showing that, for some people at least, pantothenic acid can have a real effect on the pain of arthritis. Next, we'll find out how the vitamin compares to other medications in safety and side effects, and what the right dosage for you would be. And finally, we'll talk about why the arthritis research establishment has paid almost no attention to it.

One of the goals of this book is to bring pantothenic acid to the attention of that establishment, and to get that research going again after a long delay. The other is to convince you to try pantothenic acid for your arthritis pain.

—Phyllis Eisenstein

Introduction

The Arthritis Breakthrough

This book is about a breakthrough treatment for arthritis. Some people might even call it a miracle. I did.

Twenty-four years ago, I needed a miracle. I was in so much pain from arthritis that I could barely walk, and my doctor had told me there was nothing more he could do for me. I was twenty-six years old and saw a life of misery stretching out ahead of me. I was frightened and depressed. But I didn't give up.

The pain turned me into a detective, and a combination of luck and research led me to my miracle. It turned out to be a vitamin available at my corner drugstore without a prescription, a vitamin called *pantothenic acid*. I had never heard of it, and unless you are a biochemist or a nutrition expert, you probably haven't either. But if you have arthritis, it could be your miracle, too.

If you've picked this book up, you probably already know quite a bit about arthritis. Maybe you can't open those child-proof containers anymore, or you have trouble writing anything longer than a grocery list. Maybe you grit your teeth and lean hard on the banister when you climb stairs, and you can't even imagine running to catch a bus. Maybe you can only sew, or dance, or just get through the day with the help of frequent doses of painkillers like aspirin, ibuprofen, or even the newest over-the-counter medications, naproxen sodium and ketoprofen. Or maybe you've gone past that point to the prescription pills, or to cortisone injections directly into the places that hurt.

You know how depressing arthritis can be. It's not just the pain, though sometimes the pain won't go away no matter what you take, and even lying in bed doesn't do any good. But even when the pain does go away, you know that the pills and the shots have side effects that you'd rather not think about. You've read the warnings on the labels. You've heard your doctor say you can't take cortisone too often. You know researchers are looking for a cure, but you also know they've been doing that for years and they haven't found one yet. In the meantime, you can predict changes in the weather as well as any meteorologist, and you dread the coming of rain.

Maybe you've resigned yourself to an endless round of painkillers or anti-inflammatories, and you're just hoping the side effects will stay away for a while. Or maybe you've resigned yourself to the pain, and to waiting who-knows-how-long for all that research to produce something.

But you don't have to give up, and you don't have to wait. You can learn how pantothenic acid, an inexpensive and widely available vitamin, may be able to change your life. And you can try it today.

Chapter 1

My Own Arthritis Story

Some scientists think that arthritis may be at least partly induced by stress. Maybe that was true in my case. I had certainly had a stressful year before my first attack.

I was a freshman at the University of Chicago when it happened. I had spent the summer between high school and college nursing my mother, who was in the final months of a long battle with colon cancer. When she died, just a few days before fall classes began, I was emotionally and physically exhausted. I hadn't even known for sure that I would be able to start college on time, and there I was, plunging into it almost directly after her funeral.

I was seventeen, and our family doctor had told me—with a serious hand laid on my shoulder—that I was a very strong young woman. I took that to mean he thought I could handle the tremendous changes in my life. I thought I could, too. I started school with confidence, and by midwinter, I was working harder than I ever had before, eager to make my father proud of me, and anxious to justify the high cost of tuition by earning grades good enough for the Dean's List. I didn't pay much attention to the pain in my chest at first. I assumed it was my old friend pleurisy. I had lousy tonsils and caught every respiratory bug that went around.

But I didn't have any of the other usual symptoms—no coughing, no sneezing, no sore throat or fever. There was just the pain, and in an odd place for pleurisy, in the front of the chest rather than on the side. I was living at home at the time—it was only half an hour from campus and far cheaper than the dormitory—but I didn't mention the pain to my father. He had always been too busy to deal with my illnesses; Mom and I had done that. I took some aspirin and figured I would wait it out.

Within two days, though, the pain was so bad that I was taking an aspirin every half hour, searching for the dosage that would let me breathe. Every time I tried to expand my lungs, I felt a sharp, stabbing pain in my chest. I found myself holding my breath as long as I could, then inhaling as slowly and shallowly as possible while I waited and waited for the aspirin to take hold. After twelve or fourteen aspirins, with my ears ringing and my head spinning, the pain was as bad as ever.

I'm sure I wasn't thinking straight. I didn't call my father to come home from work and help me. I didn't call our family doctor. Instead, I got on the bus and went down to the campus Student Health Service.

I must have looked terrible—I imagine I was pale and drawn, and I know I was shaking—because they took me almost immediately. The doctor who saw me was the first female doctor I had ever met, and she was very concerned. I had taken far too much aspirin, she said, and that was why my ears were ringing; I should have come in sooner. She listened to my symptoms and to my chest. Then she said, "Does this hurt?" and she poked a finger hard into the spot where one of my ribs joined my breastbone.

She took my gasp of pain as a yes.

"You have Tietze's syndrome," she said. "I'll give you a prescription for it. If you don't feel better in a week, come back. And don't take any more aspirin."

The prescription was for Darvon Compound, a combination of aspirin, caffeine, and a narcotic painkiller. In my seventeen years, I had never taken anything that strong before. It worked: it chased the pain away completely. It also made me float through the following seven days. I went to school as usual, I even got a perfect score on a French exam, though later on I couldn't quite remember actually taking the exam. But that was fine, because I didn't hurt any more. And when I was finished with my Darvon Compound, the pain didn't come back. I had been sick, but it was over, and I was back to normal—for two years.

During those years, my father died, I moved into an apartment with several other students, and I took a part-time job to make ends meet. To add to the stress, the Viet Nam War heated up and my fiancé was drafted, and I caught and recovered fairly quickly from infectious mononucleosis. Stressful times, but my grades were still good, and I was chugging along well enough.

Until January 10, 1966.

It was a bitterly cold winter evening, I remember, but I was comfortably bundled up and walking my usual mile from campus to my apartment after an afternoon in the library. About four blocks from home, my right hip began to ache. And the longer I walked, the more it ached, a bone-deep ache, nothing like a pulled muscle or some sort of bruise. After another block, the pain was a steel spike, red-hot, grinding in my hip socket. Putting weight on my right leg had become an agony, and I had to rest, canted to the left, after every step. The last three blocks to home took me more than an hour. The two flights up to my apartment were a little easier—I could lean my weight on the banister and drag myself along by my arms. I dropped my books just inside the apartment door and, clinging to doorknobs and woodwork, pulled myself into my room and fell on my bed.

One of my roommates was a student at the university's medical school and arranged for my admission to the hospital. I stayed in the hospital for five weeks, while a cluster of doctors—orthopedic surgeons and specialists from the Arthritis Clinic—puzzled over my case. I had some sort of arthritis, that was clear, but my symptoms didn't fit neatly into any of the recognized categories. Still, they were sure they could fix me.

They gave me quite a lot of aspirin, which did nothing. They injected cortisone directly into my hip socket, which did nothing. They applied wet heat to the painful area for hours every day, which did nothing. They kept me lying flat in bed for a month, only letting me sit up to use the bedpan; they said it would take the strain off the painful area and let the inflammation subside, but it did nothing. Finally, they took a series of sophisticated X-rays that showed inflammation, not in my hip, where the pain seemed to be, but in the right side of my lower back, where two of the bones—the sacrum and the ilium—met. That shouldn't have mattered, though, they said; their treatment should have helped. It was time to do something drastic, especially since my student health insurance was about to run out.

They gave me a supply of phenylbutazone pills and sent me home on crutches. I later found out that phenylbutazone was a powerful anti-inflammatory drug commonly used to take down painful inflammation in the legs of race horses. I was on the same medication given to Dancer's Image, a Kentucky Derby winner—and it was dangerous stuff. While I was taking it, I had to go back to the hospital every week for blood tests, to make sure it wasn't destroying my red blood cells. Luckily, it did its job and left my blood cells alone.

Over the next couple of weeks, the pain ebbed away, and, finally, I was able to walk normally again and discontinue the pills and tests. With great joy, I returned those crutches to the Arthritis Clinic. My only complaint was that the doctors had taken so long to find a cure for me.

Of course, it wasn't really a cure; I was fooling myself on that score. There wasn't any cure for arthritis, and I still had it. During the next six years, I had one or two attacks a year, usually in my lower back (which I still thought of as my hip), but sometimes also in my chest, and after a while in my right wrist and in the right hinge of my jaw. Arthritis, it seemed, was finding homes all over my body. But every one of them succumbed to phenylbutazone. I left school, married my fiancé (who was then in the Air Force), joined him at his base in Germany, and finally came home with him after he left the service. After hearing about my experience at the University of Chicago, Air Force doctors gave me phenylbutazone when I needed it, and so did my husband's family doctor. I thought my arthritis was under control—until February of 1972.

The attack of February 1972 was the worst I'd ever experienced. The pain was excruciating. It struck my chest, turning every breath into the stab of an ice pick, and it struck my lower back, leaving me unable to walk, unable to move around my home except by dragging myself by my arms from one piece of furniture to another. Standing on two legs was impossible, sitting down or even lying in bed was agony. I couldn't find any pain-free position. But I had faith in phenylbutazone. I called the doctor and began taking it.

It didn't work. I couldn't believe it. Phenylbutazone had always worked. It had to work.

But the days passed and passed, and nothing changed. My doctor gave me codeine for the pain, and that helped me sleep at night, and in fact it made me sleep quite a bit during the day, but it didn't let me walk. I couldn't keep taking codeine endlessly, so when it was absolutely clear that the phenylbutazone was doing nothing, my doctor sent me to an orthopedic surgeon who had a lot of experience in treating patients with arthritis.

As so many other doctors had, he ordered X-rays and peered at them for a while. Then he gave me a shot of cortisone and Xylocaine directly into the problem area.

The result was dramatic. The pain vanished. I stood up. I walked around the office. I felt great.

"That's the Xylocaine," he said. "We'll see how you are in a few hours, when it wears off. We'll see what the cortisone does. Till then, go home and lie down."

I was always a good patient; I did as he said. In fact, I went home and took a nap. When I woke up, the pain was back, as bad as ever.

Although the Xylocaine had temporarily gotten rid of my pain, using it regularly was not an option. Xylocaine, also known as lidocaine, is a local anesthetic. Dentists routinely use it to numb your mouth when they drill your teeth, and doctors use it to block pain in a variety of medical procedures. Injections of Xylocaine must be given by an expert who knows exactly where and how to give them. I certainly didn't have the expertise to give them to myself (especially not in my back) and neither did my husband, and visiting a doctor for a shot every few hours was an impossibility. Besides that, repeated doses of Xylocaine could be dangerous; the drug could build up in my body and do all sorts of bad things to me, including making me pass out, giving me convulsions, or even stopping my heart.

The doctor suggested physical therapy. So I went to the physical therapist, lay down on her table and endured a long bout of heat and massage. At the end of the session, the pain was so much worse that I couldn't get off the table, I couldn't even roll over, without her help. With great effort, I managed to hobble back to my waiting husband. I went home and phoned my doctor to report another failure.

It was 1972, and my doctor's options were more limited than they would be today. He told me there was nothing else he could give me that was better than what I had tried already. He told me I should continue to take the codeine and just learn to live with arthritis.

I hung up the phone, shocked and dismayed. Nothing else he could give me? Nothing? I didn't know what to do. My life was completely miserable. Even walking with a cane or crutches was an ordeal, because merely moving my right leg made my hip feel like someone was trying to break it off. I had visions of being in a wheelchair for the rest of my life, in pain the whole time, and a codeine addict on top of it, sleeping large chunks of my time away. I was twenty-six years old and spiraling down into a deep well of depression.

Then my husband made the suggestion that changed everything. We were both news-lovers and listened regularly to the local twenty-four-hour news radio station. Scattered among the news stories and commercials were various recorded features, one of which was a nutrition spot by Adelle Davis, who had written several books on nutritional supplements and health. What could it hurt, my husband said, to get one of her books and see what she had to say about arthritis?

We found *Let's Get Well* in paperback at a local bookstore, and I read it cover to cover. Judging from the huge list of references to reputable scientific journals in the back of the book, Ms. Davis had really done her homework, and that made me think there might be some hope in her advice. She recommended a rather large variety of supplements for arthritis, as she did for most ailments, but I was willing to give almost anything a try at that point. We went to a drug store that carried a wide selection of vitamins and minerals and bought everything she suggested. Then I started taking a handful of pills six times a day—calcium, magnesium, lecithin, vitamin A, vitamin C, vitamin D, vitamin E, and all of the B vitamins, with extra B_2, B_6, and pantothenic acid.

Within a week, I felt much better. In ten days, I was pain-free and walking normally. What could I call it but a miracle?

Had my arthritis been cured? No, because a week after I

stopped taking the pills, the pain came back. But I didn't let it escalate into unbearability this time; I restarted my supplements after the first half dozen twinges. Even so, several days passed before I felt fine again. This time, once I felt fine, I lowered my dosages instead of discontinuing them—lowered them to the maintenance level suggested in Ms. Davis's book. If the pain came back, I was supposed to return to the higher levels, otherwise, the maintenance level was intended to keep me going for the long term.

I realized then that I might be taking handfuls of supplements for the rest of my life. That didn't matter to me, of course, as long as they worked. I wasn't getting any unpleasant side effects from them, and a little library research confirmed that I wasn't taking any dangerous doses. But as I went on swallowing my pills periodically through the day, every day, I began to wonder if all of them were really necessary. Was my arthritis banished by the combination of so many different supplements, or was there one particular substance that was actually doing the job? Or maybe two?

I decided to experiment on myself. One substance at a time, I began to eliminate pills.

It took a while. I knew from discontinuing the supplements the first time that I would have to wait a week for the results on each one; obviously, whatever was working on me required that long to clear out of my system. Then I would have to double- and triple-check, trying various combinations of pills before I could be sure I had pinpointed what I was looking for. But I was patient. I kept a chart of what I was taking and when I took it. And the results were unmistakable, even after being double- and triple-checked. Pantothenic acid was the active ingredient in that handful of pills. If I stopped it, the pain came back in about a week. If I started it again, the pain went away in a few days. None of the other pills had that effect.

I discarded the rest. I stayed with pantothenic acid.

All of this happened twenty-four years ago. I've discontinued my pantothenic acid many times since then, sometimes purposely, sometimes through forgetfulness (usually while on vacation), and in every instance the pain has come back. It may have taken a week or a month, but it has always come back. And it has always gone away again, thanks to pantothenic acid.

These days there's a new place on my body that has arthritis. About a decade ago, my knee started to bother me, locking up if left in a bent position overnight or on a long plane ride, and straightening only with considerable pain. It also hurt when I climbed stairs. I had to raise my maintenance dose of pantothenic acid to take care of that. Now it is the knee that acts up first if I forget my vitamin for a few days. I try not to forget, but it's easy enough to do when I'm busy and active and feeling good.

If I don't forget, I lead a normal life, the life I thought I would never be able to go back to when my orthopedic surgeon gave up on me in 1972. I walk as much as I like, I carry my own groceries from the store to my car, and into my house. I run up and down the basement stairs to do the laundry, and I exercise on the living room floor with weights on my ankles and dumbbells in my hands. I certainly never lean on the furniture to get around, and I don't even own a cane or crutches. No one would suspect I have arthritis. In fact, when I tell people I do, they usually have trouble believing me.

I can't guarantee that pantothenic acid will work for everyone with arthritis. But I am proof that it's well worth trying. If you have arthritis, you, too, may be able to do something about your life and your health—something that won't take surgery or acupuncture or some sort of special diet in which you avoid all the foods you love.

So why don't more people know about pantothenic acid? Why didn't my doctor tell me about it? Why did I have to find out about it on my own? What is known about its connection to arthritis? How much do you have to take? And what in the world is pantothenic acid, anyway?

If you're going to do something about your arthritis, you should know what you're fighting and what your weapons are. Only then can you make an intelligent decision. So let's take a look at the enemy and at the arsenal.

Chapter 2

ARTHRITIS—THE DISEASE WITH A HUNDRED FORMS

According to the Arthritis Foundation, nearly 40 million Americans have arthritis. That's one-sixth of the total U.S. population. No wonder there are so many television commercials for arthritis pain relief products!

But what do medical scientists know about arthritis? What is it, and what parts of our bodies does it affect? How does it start, and what are its long-term consequences? In this chapter, we'll look at the answers to those questions.

We'll also discuss the major varieties of arthritis and their symptoms. If you don't already know what type of arthritis you have, this chapter can help you to identify it. If you do know, you may want to skip ahead to that section to find out more about it, and then go on to the rest of the book.

ARTHRITIS IS NOT JUST ONE THING

Most people don't know that "arthritis" is the casual, catch-all term for a whole variety of diseases—more than a hundred of them, in fact. Officially, doctors call these ailments "rheumatic diseases," and consider arthritis itself to be merely one of the major symptoms. The word *arthritis* (derived from Greek, like so many other medical terms), literally means "inflammation of a joint"—the swelling, stiffness, redness, and above all, pain that sufferers know so well. Yet there are degrees and varieties of arthritis, so that one person's arthritis can be quite different from another's in the area affected, the level of pain, and the amount of damage done. Arthritis can be associated with diseases we don't ordinarily think of as affecting joints, such as psoriasis or Lyme disease. Or it can be the main problem itself, as with osteoarthritis and rheumatoid arthritis. Arthritis can strike once and then vanish, it can become a periodic visitor, or it can settle in as a permanent companion. And one person can have different forms of arthritis at different times, or even at the same time.

The first thing we have to do, if we want to understand anything about arthritis, is to understand where arthritis strikes.

THE AFFECTED AREA: THE JOINT

A joint is a place where two (or more) bones come together. Joints are the working areas of the body, the places where the most physical stress occurs. There are three kinds of joints, only two of which are affected by arthritis. The third kind, the *fixed joint*, occurs between the bony plates of a child's skull and allows the skull to expand as the child's growing brain expands; when the brain stops growing, in adolescence, these joints become solid bone and are no longer flexible. The other two kinds of joints, the ones where arthritis can strike, are supposed to remain flexible throughout life. These are the *cartilaginous joints* and the *synovial joints*.

The cartilaginous joints are the less flexible of the two. Because joints are places where hard and unyielding bones must move against each other, there has to be some kind of cushioning material present, or else the surface of the bone would scratch, pit, and wear away from friction. One such material is *cartilage,* an elastic, spongelike substance that, in cartilaginous joints, covers and protects the parts of the bones that would otherwise rub. Your spine is a set of cartilaginous joints piled one on top of another, an alternating column of bone and cartilage that extends from your hips to your head. The bones are called vertebrae, and each piece of cartilage is called a disc. When you have a slipped disc, it is one of these pieces of cartilage that is out of place.

Other cartilaginous joints occur in the pelvis, where they allow slight movements at the front (between the two pubic bones) and at the back (the *sacroiliac joint,* where the bottom section of the spine meets the hipbone). The ends of the ribs at the front of your chest are also connected to each other and to the breastbone by cartilage.

The more flexible joints are called synovial joints: the shoulders, hips, elbows, knees, wrists, ankles, fingers, and toes. Moving far more than the cartilaginous joints, they are subject to more wear and tear, and they need even more cushioning. The bone ends in these joints are also covered with protective cartilage, but in addition, they are cushioned by the *synovium,* a thin membrane containing a viscous fluid (synovial fluid) that acts as a lubricant. This synovial fluid does the same job in your body that oil does in your car.

In order to work properly, though, these very mobile synovial joints need more than cushioning. The bone ends need to be kept aligned with each other. This is accomplished partly through the shapes of the bone ends themselves, the curves of one bony surface neatly fitting and moving against those of the other. But mainly, the bones stay in correct alignment because they are surrounded by the soft tissues of ligaments, tendons, and muscles.

Ligaments are fibrous bands that attach to the bones, hold them together, and keep them from shifting out of place or from moving in directions that can damage them. The ligaments on either side of your finger joints, for example, prevent the fingers from bending side-to-side, a motion that those joints are not constructed for and not cushioned to withstand. Muscles make the bones move, and they are connected to those bones by tendons, which are dense, tough, fibrous cords that can withstand the considerable pull of those muscles. Like ligaments, muscles and tendons also help to keep the bones from moving in the wrong ways. There are no ligaments in your shoulder—ligaments would prevent its wide range of motion—but tendons and small muscles are enough to keep the end of the upper arm bone from slipping out of its socket.

Like the bones, the ligaments, tendons, and muscles also need protection against the wear and tear of friction. So where friction would occur, where the ligaments, tendons, and muscles cross and slide upon bones or other muscles, they are cushioned by small sacs filled with synovial fluid. Since these crossings and slidings occur frequently around joints, such sacs—called *bursas*—are found there.

Bursas round out our picture of a joint, which is, of course, something far more complicated than just a place where two (or more) bones come together. A joint is, rather, a machine that is supposed to work smoothly, moved by muscles, lubricated by synovial fluid, cushioned and held together by various soft tissues. But like any machine, it sometimes breaks down.

WHAT DO WE KNOW ABOUT ARTHRITIS?

Scientists are still struggling to understand the causes of arthritis. A few forms appear to be caused—or at least triggered—by old injuries or infections, but the current medical thought is that, in general, arthritis is an immune response gone wrong. Normally, the body's immune system fights invaders (antigens) such as bacteria and viruses with specialized substances (antibodies) that also cause inflammation of the body's own tissues. This is, for example, the source of the rash you get during a measles infection. After the invaders are destroyed, these substances stop being manufactured and the inflammation subsides. In arthritis, the immune system is fighting in the same way, and producing inflammation, but there are no invaders present. Many scientists think that under these circumstances the immune system must be misidentifying its own body's cells as invaders, and attacking them. This would make arthritis an autoimmune disease ("auto" meaning "self"). But so far, nobody knows exactly how this happens, or why.

Quite a lot, however, is known about the various symptoms of the one hundred-odd forms of rheumatic disease, about the specific parts of the body they affect, and about the damage they do. Although the American College of Rheumatologists lists ten categories of rheumatic diseases, the most common of them can be grouped into three broad classes; osteoarthritis, inflammatory arthritis, and extra-articular disorders. And, even though only one of these categories is called "inflammatory," they all involve inflammation to some extent, and affect the joints or the tissues surrounding the joints.

Let's look at some of these diseases in order to achieve a better understanding of what they are and what they do. Perhaps you'll recognize your own form of arthritis among them.

OSTEOARTHRITIS

Osteoarthritis, also known as "degenerative joint disease," is the most common form of arthritis, affecting nearly half of the people who are identified as having arthritis. Rare in children and young adults, it is often considered a natural and inevitable result of aging, even though many elderly people do not suffer from it. It is a disease that develops slowly, usually over the course of years.

At the beginning, a person with osteoarthritis experiences joint pain following vigorous activity, and stiffness the next morning, but a good night's rest gets rid of the pain, and a few minutes of flexing and stretching banishes the stiffness. Later, the more ordinary activities of life start causing pain, and as time goes on, smaller and smaller movements do it. Eventually, every little motion is painful, even resting quietly may hurt, and sleep becomes difficult because of that. The joints may feel like they are cracking or grating whenever they move, and they may enlarge and become less movable. The pain may radiate from the affected joint—across the shoulders and down the arms, for example, if the arthritic area is in the neck, or into the groin and buttocks and down the inside of the thigh, even as far as the knee, if the affected joint is the hip.

"Degenerative joint disease" is a good description of what is going on inside an osteoarthritic joint. Gradually, over time, the cartilage that cushions the joint disintegrates, exposing the underlying bones to friction as the joint continues to be used. The bone responds to the wear from friction by trying to rebuild itself, but the process of rebuilding doesn't work very well and results in thickened and uneven surfaces that are full of bone spurs. The larger and rougher bony ends no longer move properly against each other, limiting the motion of the joint; they also irritate the surrounding soft tissues and cause inflammation. After a while, the muscles around the painful area can become weak and begin to atrophy from lack of use.

The joints most commonly affected by osteoarthritis are the fingers, hips, knees, neck, and lower spine.

Doctors divide osteoarthritis into two categories, not according to which joints are affected, but according to whether or not some cause for the disease is known. In primary osteoarthritis, no cause is known; it just happens. In secondary osteoarthritis, the cause is known—or at least presumed—to be some other disease (such as rheumatoid arthritis or gout) or some injury. A joint that has already been badly damaged, as in a sports accident, is likely to develop osteoarthritis later on. So is a joint subjected to the kinds of repetitive on-the-job physical stress that jackhammer operators, riveters, and ballet dancers experience. But beyond these fairly obvious factors, the causes of osteoarthritis are hazy and uncertain. Obesity—presumably another source of repetitive physical stress—seems to have an association with osteoarthritis of the knee but not, as might be expected, with osteoarthritis of the hip, which is also stressed in holding the obese body up. There are some cases of osteoarthritis in which hereditary factors appear to be involved. Hormones also may play a role, because postmenopausal women who take estrogen seem to have a lower incidence of osteoarthritis than those who don't. But the question of why people who injure a joint often don't develop osteoarthritis in it until many years later has yet to be answered.

Recently, some experts have suggested that the reason they can't find a cause for primary osteoarthritis is that it may not be a single disease but rather a group of diseases, with the same results coming from different causes.

INFLAMMATORY ARTHRITIS

The category of inflammatory arthritis includes the other most commonly occurring forms of arthritis—rheumatoid arthritis, gout, ankylosing spondylitis, arthritis associated with systemic lupus erythematosus, and infectious arthritis.

Rheumatoid Arthritis

Rheumatoid arthritis is the second most common form of arthritis, and one of the most crippling; somewhere between two-and-one-half and five million Americans suffer from it, and it strikes young and middle-aged people as well as old. In most people it starts subtly, with a generalized tired, achy feeling, almost like the flu, that can last for weeks or months before the real joint pain begins. Once the pain does begin, several joints are usually affected at the same time, becoming swollen, red, and warm to the touch, and, of course, tender.

Attacks of rheumatoid arthritis tend to be episodic, though unpredictable in length; they might last weeks or months, then fade away for a comparable time before coming back. During an attack (or *flare*, as doctors call it), the pain may be constant, even when the sufferer lies completely still, and stiffness may also be constant, though it more typically lasts only for an hour or so after a night's sleep. Daytime fatigue continues all through the flare.

Over time, with continuing flares, other symptoms crop up. The affected joints may gradually become deformed, a process most obvious in the fingers, which may become permanently bent in unnatural positions. Joints may lose their mobility and become frozen in place—this is especially common in the shoulder. Other parts of the body besides the joints may show the visible effects of rheumatoid arthritis: fleshy nodules may appear under the skin, often on the forearm or at the Achilles tendon; the eyes may become dry and inflamed; sores that refuse to heal may appear on the legs; and the lymph nodes may become swollen.

Inside the body, where medical tests can find it, much more is going on. Scientists consider rheumatoid arthritis a systemic disease—not a disease limited to the joints, but one that affects the whole body. It is definitely recognized as an autoimmune disorder, but as with so many other forms of arthritis, its ultimate cause is not known. About 85 percent of patients with rheumatoid arthritis have a particular antibody in their blood, called *rheumatoid factor*, but what the presence of that factor really means is unknown, because people with quite a few other diseases, including tuberculosis, rubella, influenza, and periodontal disease also have it. What *is* known is that rheumatoid arthritis is a connective tissue disease, and that is why it affects so many different parts of the body.

Connective tissue is the material that supports our bodies, holds them together, and gives them shape. Bone, cartilage, tendons, and ligaments are all connective tissue, as are the walls of our veins and arteries, the sheaths that enclose our muscles and internal organs, and the true skin (the *dermis*), that underlies the outer layer we can see (the *epidermis*). The synovium, too, is made of connective tissue, and inflammation of the synovium is the initial cause of the joint pain of rheumatoid arthritis. As the disease progresses, the synovium gradually changes from its normal form to one that induces the body to eat away at its own cartilage, bone, and soft tissue. Tendons that become irritated and inflamed in this process may shorten, immobilizing the joint as a splint would, and giving the damaged, no-longer-cushioned ends of the bones an opportunity to fuse together and become rigid. Or, the tendons may tear, leaving the joint loose and wobbly. Outside the joints, the inflammation of rheumatoid arthritis can affect the skin, the eyes, the nerves, the heart, the lungs, the blood vessels, and the spleen. It can impair circulation to the hands and feet. The disease almost always causes anemia. And perhaps the most chilling scientific observation of all is that people with severe rheumatoid arthritis appear to die ten to fifteen years earlier than expected of infections, lung and kidney diseases, and gastrointestinal bleeding.

The joints that may be affected by rheumatoid arthritis are those in the jaw, neck, shoulder, elbow, hand, hip, knee, ankle, and foot.

Gout

Gout, affecting between one and two-and-one-half million Americans, is the most common form of inflammatory arthritis among men over thirty, and probably the second most common form of inflammatory arthritis overall. It usually appears suddenly, often developing overnight, making a single joint swollen, red, warm, and so tender that the sufferer can't bear the weight of a blanket on it. Early attacks tend to last three to ten days and then subside, leaving the person pain free for long periods; later attacks may be more frequent, last longer, and involve more joints. Eventually, the affected joints may become deformed.

The accepted reason for the inflammation of gout is the presence of crystals of sodium urate in the joint. We all have countless substances dissolved in our blood and other body fluids, but people with gout have unusually high levels of urate in their blood, and the excess can form crystals in various parts of the body, including the joints and the urinary tract. Yet the connection between high urate levels and gout is not really quite that clear, because the majority of people with high levels of urate in their blood, and even urate crystals in their joints, never develop gout at all. And in people with gout, urate crystals are sometimes found in joints that are not inflamed. As with arthritis in general, much research remains to be done on gout.

Although the knee, ankle, foot, or hand may be affected, gout seems to have a strong preference for the joint at the base of the big toe. If uncontrolled, gout can lead to destruction of the cartilage and bone of the affected joints, causing those joints to become deformed. A person with uncontrolled gout may also develop kidney stones made of those urate crystals; in some cases, the stones may even have formed before the first attack of joint pain, or they may even be the person's only symptom of gout. (There are, however, other kinds of kidney stones that have no connection to gout.)

Ankylosing Spondylitis and Its Relatives

Ankylosing spondylitis is one of a group of related rheumatic diseases called seronegative spondylarthropathies, a name that means that the people who suffer from these ailments do not have rheumatoid factor in their blood ("seronegative") but do show joint disease of the spine ("spondylarthropathy"). About two million Americans have these spondylarthropathies, some three hundred thousand with ankylosing spondylitis itself.

The symptoms of ankylosing spondylitis usually begin in adolescence or early adulthood, the most common one being a dull, low-back pain. Back stiffness, with or without pain, is another common early symptom, as is pain in a hip or shoulder. Or there may be tenderness along various bones, near but not in joints, or chest pain upon coughing, sneezing, or even just deep breathing. The stiffness is usually worst in the morning, easing up with a hot shower and mild physical activity. The pain may come and go at first, but within a few months it becomes constant. Long periods of inactivity, as well as cold, damp weather, make both pain and stiffness worse.

Over a period of ten years or more, the spine can become increasingly stiff, severely limiting movement; if the neck is affected, for example, the person may no longer be able to turn his head without turning his whole body. The spine may even stiffen in a bent position, especially if the sufferer is not careful about exercising and maintaining good posture. Pain and deformity in a hip may eventually be so extreme that it requires hip replacement. In addition, more than a quarter of those who have ankylosing spondylitis experience bouts of acute uveitis, a painful eye inflammation. And after many years of the disease, a small number of individuals can have heart and lung problems.

Although it can cause inflammation of the hips and shoulders, which are synovial joints, ankylosing spondylitis is mainly a disease of the cartilaginous joints and of the places where ligaments and tendons attach to the bones (the *entheses*). "Ankylosing" means "crooked" or "bent" and refers to the bending that can happen to the spine over the course of time. The inflammation caused by the disease roughens the surface of the bone, stimulating it to repair itself. But the repair process is overenthusiastic and produces bone that grows beyond the original surface, into the soft tissue of the cartilage, ligaments, or tendons. This continues until the soft tissue has actually been replaced by bone ("ossified"), and the bones are fused together and no longer flexible. The rigid spine, in addition to limiting a person's mobility, is also vulnerable to fracture in relatively minor accidents, and such fractures can injure the spinal cord.

The other seronegative spondylarthropathies can also affect the spine, but their true common symptoms are their inflammatory effect on the entheses and their association with various other, non-arthritis ailments. It is these non-arthritis diseases that differentiate the spondylarthropathies from each other. *Reiter's syndrome,* for example, is preceded by diarrhea and urinary tract inflammation due to bacterial infection. *Psoriatic arthritis* occurs in people with the skin disease psoriasis. *Enteropathic arthritis* accompanies various non-infectious digestive tract diseases such as ulcerative colitis and Crohn's disease. *Reactive arthritis* occurs after digestive tract or sexually transmitted infections such as those caused by Salmonella or Chlamydia. In none of these cases, though, does having the other disease guarantee that the individual will develop the spondylarthropathy. For example, psoriatic arthritis occurs in only 5 to 7 percent of people with psoriasis.

Reiter's syndrome, psoriatic arthritis, and enteropathic arthritis can all cause the swelling and deformity in the hands known as "sausage digits," named from the sausage-like appearance of the fingers. Psoriatic arthritis produces joint damage that resembles rheumatoid arthritis, while the damage of Reiter's syndrome, enteropathic arthritis, and reactive arthritis are similar to that of ankylosing spondylitis. All of the spondylarthropathies can be recurring, long-lasting, and even disabling.

Systemic Lupus Erythematosus (SLE)

SLE affects about one hundred twenty five thousand people in the U.S., and the vast majority of them are women. Like rheumatoid arthritis, SLE is considered an autoimmune disease, and its cause is unknown, though it appears to run in families. Also like rheumatoid arthritis, it is a disease of the connective tissue. Of the many symptoms associated with it, the most obvious is a butterfly-shaped skin rash across the bridge of the nose and both cheeks, although SLE can also cause rashes, and even lumpy swellings, thick scaling, and scarring in other skin areas. Other symptoms include fever, overwhelming fatigue, and weight loss. There may also be headaches, abdominal pain and nausea, pneumonia, and even chest pain. Many of these symptoms are due to inflammation; for example, the abdominal pain is usually caused by inflammation of the membrane that encloses the intestines, and the chest pain by inflammation of the membrane that surrounds the heart. Inflammation also causes one of the most common symptoms of SLE, arthritis.

Any joint may be involved in this form of arthritis, but the hands, wrists, and knees are the usual sites of pain. Unlike rheumatoid arthritis, this variety does not usually damage the bones themselves, but swelling of the synovium and other soft tissue around the joints can pull those joints out of their normal alignment, causing permanent deformity, especially in the fingers, which can bend toward the outside edge of the hand (the side where the little finger is), or can take on a backward-bent, arched appearance called a "swan neck."

SLE can do serious damage to the kidneys, heart, lungs, blood vessels, and nervous system.

Infectious Arthritis

Bacteria, viruses, fungi, and other microscopic organisms can cause arthritis if they reach the joints. There, they can trigger the body's immune response, provoking inflammation of the synovium and other surrounding soft tissues simply because they are outside invaders. They can also directly damage bone and cartilage by producing various destructive chemicals. This form of arthritis may be temporary if the underlying ailment can be cured promptly (for example, antibiotics for a bacterial infection). But if there is no cure, or if treatment is delayed too long, the arthritis can become a permanent condition, cartilage and bone can erode away, and the joints can become deformed.

Infectious arthritis can accompany almost any kind of infection, including those from wounds, surgery, intravenous needle use, and diseases of the lungs, urinary tract, or digestive tract. It can also be brought on by gonorrhea, hepatitis B, human parvovirus (which can cause fifth disease), human immunodeficiency virus (HIV), rubella (German measles), syphilis, tuberculosis, leprosy, and brucellosis (Mediterranean fever, Malta fever, or undulant fever).

Lyme disease, caused by a microscopic organism spread by tick bites, results in arthritis in about 60 percent of its victims. The joints affected are the large ones, especially the knees. Antibiotics, which kill the micro-organism, usually (but not always) get rid of the arthritis.

EXTRA-ARTICULAR DISORDERS

The extra-articular ("outside the joints") disorders are a group of ailments that involve inflammation of soft tissues that are not within the joints themselves, though they are nearby.

Tendinitis and Bursitis

Tendinitis and bursitis are the most commonly occurring members of this group, and unlike other rheumatic diseases, their direct causes can often be found. Either a single sudden injury or a long period of repeated overuse, especially when the affected area has been in an abnormal body position, can cause the painful inflammation of a tendon, ligament, or bursa.

Rotator cuff tendinitis, in which a tendon that helps to hold the shoulder in place becomes inflamed, is the most common cause of shoulder pain; it is usually caused by too much overhead use of the arm. Tennis elbow, golfer's elbow, and jumper's knee are all common forms of tendinitis, caused by overuse, as is carpal tunnel syndrome, probably the most familiar of all the extra-articular disorders.

The carpal tunnel is a narrow passage inside the wrist, formed by the wrist bones (on three sides) and a ligament (on the fourth side). An important nerve and several tendons pass through this tunnel, and if any of the tissues that surround the nerve press on it (for example, if one of the tendons swells up), the parts of the hand that are fed by that nerve can either hurt or go numb. The tendons can, of course, swell up from overuse while in a single limited position, as computer keyboard users so often discover.

The pain of tendinitis or bursitis can hang on for a very long time, or if it goes away, it may recur later. Sometimes the affected area undergoes calcification. This is a process in which crystals of some of the calcium salts that are normally dissolved in our body fluids are slowly deposited in the soft tissue. These crystals do not make the soft tissue itself hard, but they do form hard little clumps embedded in the soft tissue. Unlike gout sufferers, people who experience calcification of damaged tissue do not have unusually high levels of the associated calcium salts in their blood. Rather, scientists believe that a number of different factors can cause these crystals to deposit, including age, disease, or the physical and chemical activity (or lack of it) of the damaged tissue itself. Calcification is particularly common in the shoulder, and the presence of these calcium crystals can cause further attacks of painful inflammation.

Fibromyalgia

Fibromyalgia is probably the most controversial and least understood of all rheumatic diseases. It is a cluster of symptoms without any known underlying cause. There is no inflammation or bone damage associated with the disease. Tests that help identify different kinds of arthritis, such as X-rays or blood tests, show nothing significant in fibromyalgia sufferers. Yet the pain of fibromyalgia is real.

Found in about 15 percent of patients who visit arthritis specialists, fibromyalgia occurs more often in women than in men. Its most common symptoms are fatigue and a generalized achiness, as well as pain somewhere in the neck, the chest, or the upper or lower back, frequently accompanied by morning stiffness. Also common are irritable bowel syndrome (in nearly half of fibromyalgia cases), tension headaches, a tingling and prickling of the hands and arms, and a sensation of the hands being swollen even though they don't look swollen. The person with fibromyalgia is also likely to sleep poorly. The diagnosis of fibromyalgia is confirmed if, in addition to widespread pain, there are specific places on the body that are tender to a hard poke with a finger. These include spots at the base of the skull, around the neck and shoulders, just above and just below the buttocks, just below the insides of the elbows, and on the kneecaps. And all of these symptoms may be aggravated by flares of any other forms of arthritis that the fibromyalgia sufferer may have.

Fibromyalgia does not cause any joint deformity.

OTHERS

Although some of the less common rheumatic diseases also fit into the above three groups, many of them do not. For example, Tietze's syndrome, which is an inflammation of the cartilage connecting the ribs to the breastbone, doesn't. Nor does sarcoidosis, which is primarily a lung problem though, in 10 to 15 percent of the people who have it, this condition also involves arthritis; or Charcot joint, a joint inflammation that can lead to joint destruction and loss of deep pain sensation; or palindromic rheumatism, which mounts sudden, brief periodic attacks and, over time, can evolve into rheumatoid arthritis; or arthritis caused by tumors, errors of metabolism, diabetes, thyroid disease, hemophilia, sickle cell anemia, or leukemia, and many more. So, scientists who place the major forms of rheumatic disease into the three broad categories described above add a fourth—miscellaneous—to cover the leftovers.

How Many Categories Are There, Really?

In fact, the process of classifying the hundred-odd rheumatic diseases has been going on for decades, with the categories constantly shifting and changing as researchers have found out more and more about these ailments. The three-plus-one category system above is just one of several recent schemes for classifying rheumatic diseases. The American College of Rheumatologists (ACR) uses a system of ten categories. *The Primer on the Rheumatic Diseases* (1993), published by the Arthritis Foundation, doesn't offer broad categories at all, but has one chapter on each of forty-five groups of rheumatic diseases.

To make matters more confusing, how any individual disease is classified varies from one system to another. For example, the ten-category ACR scheme places Tietze's syndrome (pain and inflammation in the cartilage where the ribs join the breastbone) in a class called "Bone and Cartilage Disorders," along with osteoporosis (loss of bone mass) and caisson disease (joint pain caused by sudden lowering of high air pressure; also known as "the bends"), and says it is merely another name for costochondritis (pain, without inflammation, in the cartilage where the ribs join the breast bone). *The Primer* places it among "Regional Rheumatic Pain Syndromes," along with tendinitis and carpal tunnel syndrome, and says it is a separate disease from costochondritis, though very similar to it.

What these wildly different classification systems really mean is that medical science still doesn't understand rheumatic diseases very well. In spite of that, doctors have some kind of treatment for every one of those hundred-odd ailments. In the next chapter we'll look at some of the most widely-used treatments and see what they do to arthritis and to the people who have that arthritis.

Chapter 3

THE STANDARD TREATMENTS

There are many different kinds of treatments for arthritis. Which one will work best for you depends on what variety of arthritis you have, how severe your symptoms are, what side effects you experience from any particular treatment, and how well you tolerate them. We are all individuals, with our own individual ways of reacting to medication. A drug that works well for one person may fail for another. It may have no side effects at all in one person and such bad ones in another that it has to be discontinued.

In this chapter, we will look at these standard treatments for arthritis and alert you to those unwanted, unpleasant, and sometimes life-threatening side effects.

ANTIBIOTICS

Because infectious arthritis and Lyme disease are infections, they are treated with antibiotics.

Infections are caused by micro-organisms, such as bacteria and viruses, that are so small that individual ones can only be seen under a microscope. These micro-organisms are usually introduced into our bodies from the outside and multiply wildly inside us until they make us sick. (A few infections are caused by micro-organisms that normally live quietly in our bodies but just get out of control). They vary in intensity and danger from the trivial, like the common cold, to the life-threatening, like bubonic plague. You've probably had countless infections in your lifetime. We are able to fight off some of these infections with our body's own natural defenses, but others require outside help. To combat them, medical scientists have developed a wide range of antibiotics.

An antibiotic is a chemical substance produced by one micro-organism to destroy another micro-organism. An example of such a substance is penicillin, which is made by a green mold and is very effective in destroying a number of different kinds of bacterial infections, including strep throat, pneumonia, spinal meningitis, and diphtheria. There are many different types of antibiotics, and each is effective against some micro-organisms and not against others. Those that can kill a lot of different ones are called broad-spectrum antibiotics; those that kill only a few kinds are called narrow-spectrum.

Not every infection will succumb to antibiotic treatment, but infectious arthritis and Lyme disease usually will. Infectious arthritis can be caused by a number of different micro-organisms, and so the antibiotic used to combat it will depend on exactly which one. In Lyme disease, which is caused by one particular micro-organism, the medications of choice are amoxicillin or doxycycline, both broad-spectrum antibiotics. In both infectious arthritis and Lyme disease, the antibiotics are given for periods of time ranging from ten to thirty days, depending on the severity of the infection. The side effects of antibiotics can include diarrhea, nausea, vomiting, skin rashes, and, in women, vaginal yeast infections.

ORAL ANALGESICS

A number of medications that do nothing other than relieve pain are sometimes used for arthritis. Of these, acetaminophen (Tylenol, Anacin-3, etc.) is available without a prescription, and pentazocine (Talwin), propoxyphene (Darvon), and codeine must be prescribed by a doctor.

Acetaminophen is the least potent of the lot, though it does relieve minor pain and is frequently useful in osteoarthritis. Its possible side effects include nausea, vomiting, diarrhea, jaundice, rash, and tiredness.

Pentazocine, propoxyphene, and codeine are all strong analgesics that can produce drug dependence. In addition, they may cause lightheadedness, dizziness, drowsiness, nausea, and vomiting.

TOPICAL ANALGESICS

A large number of pain relief creams, lotions, sprays, gels, and patches whose labels say they can be used for arthritis are available at your local drug store without a prescription. They may contain methyl salicylate, trolamine salicylate, menthol, camphor, capsaicin, or any combination of those ingredients. They may even contain ammonia. The salicylates are related to aspirin, they affect pain and inflammation in much the same way that aspirin does, and can have similar side effects (see NSAIDs, below). If you use them along with oral aspirin, you may well be overdosing. The other substances just kill pain without affecting inflammation, and they can be used along with oral medication. The most common side effect of all these products is skin irritation, especially if the skin is already irritated or broken.

NON-STEROIDAL ANTI-INFLAMMATORY DRUGS (NSAIDS)

The NSAIDs—Non-Steroidal Anti-Inflammatory Drugs—are by far the most common medications used to treat rheumatic diseases. You can buy some of them over the counter at your local drug store or supermarket: aspirin, ibuprofen, naproxen sodium (Aleve), and ketoprofen (Orudis KT). Others, like indomethacin (Indocin), diclofenac (Voltaren, Cataflam), piroxicam (Feldene), oxaprozin (Daypro), and many more, require a prescription. They all act quickly to reduce pain and inflammation, but they only last a short time. Once they are flushed completely out of the body, which takes from a few hours to a few days, depending on the drug, the arthritis symptoms return. So NSAIDs have to be taken regularly, some just once a day, some two, three, four, or even six times a day, and for long periods of time, since flares of arthritis can last for weeks or months. This is plenty of time for the side effects of these drugs to show up.

As a group, the NSAIDs have many side effects in common. They tend to irritate the stomach and may cause pain, heartburn, and indigestion. If you have an ulcer, they may make it worse; if you don't, they may give you one. They can cause abdominal cramps, gas, nausea, vomiting, diarrhea, constipation, or urinary tract irritation; rashes, headaches, blurred vision, ulcers in the mouth, or ringing in the ears. They may make you dizzy or drowsy or tired, depressed or nervous. They may make you retain fluid and gain weight or be anorexic and lose weight. If you already have kidney trouble, they may make it worse. And in high doses over a long period of time, they may cause kidney or liver damage.

One NSAID, phenylbutazone, has the potential to be so toxic to the liver and the bone marrow that it is prescribed only as a last resort these days, and is no longer even listed in the *Physicians' Desk Reference* of prescription drugs.

NSAIDs do reduce pain and inflammation, but they do

not have any effect on the underlying disease. Thus, the damage to the joints and other organs may continue in spite of the medication. Because of their side effects, some doctors try to wean their patients off of NSAIDs, substituting acetaminophen when possible.

CORTICOSTEROIDS

The natural corticosteroids, including cortisone, are hormones manufactured in the adrenal gland, a small organ located on top of the kidney. In our bodies, they are involved in sugar production in the liver and in maintaining proper sugar levels in the blood. In the 1940s, it was discovered that large doses of cortisone could dramatically reduce the inflammation of arthritis. It seemed a miracle at the time, but unfortunately, the side effects of such large doses turned out to be substantial. As a result, synthetic corticosteroids like prednisone and methylprednisone were developed that worked as well on inflammation but had less extreme side effects.

Even so, the side effects of long-term synthetic corticosteroid use, even at low doses, can be unpleasant and even health-threatening. The least serious of them include growth of facial hair, acne, fluid retention, weight gain, easy bruising, sleeplessness, muscle wasting, and headaches. More serious are stomach ulcers, inflammation of the pancreas, and the leaching of calcium from the bones (osteoporosis), which makes fracturing easier. Because synthetic corticosteroids suppress the immune response, they increase the risk of bacterial infections (which the immune response would fight) and slow or even prevent wound healing. They can promote narrowing of the blood vessels by fatty deposits and calcification (atherosclerosis). They can cause cataracts and glaucoma. And, they can also suppress the normal function of the adrenal glands, making it impossible for those glands to produce their natural hormones when the body needs them to respond to the stress of injury, infection, or surgery; this can lead to weakness and even make a person collapse.

High doses of corticosteroids can spread previously limited infections to all parts of the body, they can actually kill the living parts of bone (ultimately making the bone collapse), and they can cause perforations of the bowel. People have even died after high intravenous doses of corticosteroids.

SLOW-ACTING ANTI-RHEUMATIC DRUGS (SAARDS)

These drugs are actually known by two names—Slow-Acting Anti-Rheumatic Drugs, or SAARDs, and Disease-Modifying Anti-Rheumatic Drugs, or DMARDs. As the first name indicates, these drugs take a long time to get going, but eventually they do have an effect on the diseases they are used to treat. They are primarily used to treat the inflammatory kinds of arthritis, especially rheumatoid arthritis, ankylosing spondylitis, and arthritis associated with systemic lupus erythematosus.

Antimalarials

Although chloroquine (Aralen) and hydroxychloroquine (Plaquenil) were originally developed for use against malaria, both have been used to treat connective tissue diseases since the 1950s. Their side effects include indigestion, nausea, vomiting, headaches, nervousness, diarrhea, abdominal cramps, psoriasis, ringing in the ears, and blurred vision. The risk of eye damage is great enough that doctors recommend an eye examination every six months for anyone taking these drugs.

D-penicillamine

More than a quarter of the patients who take D-penicillamine (Cuprimine) quit within a year because of the side effects. These include nausea, vomiting, diarrhea, rashes, kidney damage, blood abnormalities, drug-induced lupus, and even myasthenia gravis (a disease in which the muscles of your body gradually become weaker and weaker). People who take D-penicillamine need to have regular blood and urine tests to determine whether they should stay on the drug.

Sulfasalazine

About half the people who take sulfasalazine (Azulfidine) develop side effects, mostly within the first four months of treatment. Rashes, nausea, vomiting, abdominal pain, headaches, and blood and liver abnormalities are the common ones. In addition, anyone who is allergic to sulfa will be allergic to sulfasalazine. People taking this drug need to have regular blood and liver tests.

Gold

The side effects of gold therapy are the major reason why people give up on it. Nearly half of the people who are treated with gold compounds experience diarrhea, and other side effects include indigestion, gas, nausea, abdominal pain, loss of appetite, ulcers in the mouth, rashes, itching, conjunctivitis, kidney problems, blood abnormalities, and upper respiratory inflammation. Injected gold (Myochrisine, Solganol) seems to be more effective against arthritis than gold taken by mouth (Ridaura), but its side effects are worse.

People taking these drugs, especially those on injected gold, must be monitored very carefully for blood and kidney damage with regular blood and urine tests.

Methotrexate

Methotrexate (Rheumatrex) works faster than most of the other SAARDs. Its most common side effects are nausea and loss of appetite, especially in the twenty-four hours following administration of the drug, but it can also cause abdominal pain, rashes, anemia, ulcers, headaches, drowsiness, blurred vision, lung damage, fibrosis or cirrhosis of the liver, urinary tract irritation, and kidney damage. People taking this drug need to have regular blood and liver tests.

Cyclosporin

The majority of people who take cyclosporin (Sandimmune) experience decreased kidney function and elevated blood pressure. It can also cause headaches, gum swelling, tremors, and convulsions. People taking it need to have regular blood and blood pressure tests.

Azathioprine

Azathioprine (Imuran) is slightly more likely to produce side effects than other SAARDs. Nausea, vomiting, and diarrhea are the most common, with bone marrow suppression and hepatitis less so. People taking this drug need to have regular blood and liver tests.

With long-term use, there is an increased risk of cancer.

Alkylating Agents

The major side effect of these drugs—chlorambucil (Leukeran) and cyclophosphamide (Cytoxan)—is an increased risk of cancer. Chlorambucil can also cause nausea, vomiting, diarrhea, mouth sores, and blood abnormalities. Cyclophosphamide can also cause urinary tract bleeding, a higher risk of infection with shingles, and infertility. As with so many other SAARDs, the use of these drugs requires regular blood tests, and cyclophosphamide also requires regular urine tests.

ANTI-RHEUMATIC DRUGS: AN OVERVIEW

It doesn't look good. Everywhere you turn, the side effects loom, and they loom larger the more powerful the drug, the longer you take it, and the larger the dose. Headache, diarrhea, nausea, ulcers, kidney damage . . . cancer? Sure, the doctor will say there's only a chance you'll experience the side effects; lots of people don't. For NSAIDs, the frequency of side effects ranges from one to twenty percent, depending on the particular drug and the particular side effect. For some of the SAARDs (gold, D-penicillamine, and sulfasalazine), the frequency of side effects is much higher. For others, it is uncertain, although those side effects are serious enough, and have been observed often enough, for the drug companies to warn doctors about them.

Many of the more minor side effects, like headache, nausea, dizziness, and drowsiness, will disappear quickly once you stop taking the drug that is causing them. Others, like skin rashes and diarrhea, may take a little longer. Vaginal yeast infections won't go away by themselves at all, and must be treated with yeast-killing medication. Of the more serious side effects, suppression of the adrenal glands can last for months after corticosteroids have been stopped. Kidney and liver damage, if caught early enough, are completely reversible once you stop taking the drug that caused them (these organs will heal themselves), but if the damage has gone too far, it will be permanent. Other side effects, like osteoporosis, atherosclerosis, cataracts, or cancer, don't go away just because you stop the anti-rheumatic drugs.

As with all medications, you and your doctor have to weigh the potential benefits of these drugs against their potential risks. Many people take ibuprofen, for example, for years without any trouble at all. Maybe you'll be one of those.

But in case you're not, or in case you don't want to take that chance, what other options are there?

NON-DRUG APPROACHES

Doctors tend to take a pharmaceutical approach to arthritis, but there are a number of other proven approaches that don't involve drugs. In general, these are non-toxic, non-invasive, and relatively inexpensive, and their results are easy to judge. Some you can even do for yourself at home.

Rest

Because fatigue can so often intensify the discomfort of arthritis, and because rest can actually reduce inflammation and relieve pain, it is important to get enough rest. Sometimes this means taking a nap in the middle of the day, in addition to a full night's sleep, especially during flares. Often, just lying down for a little while a few times a day is helpful. For people who work full-time, spending a coffee break or part of lunch lying down can help (on a couch or even on a folding foam mat you bring with you from home, set in an out-of-the-way place). Yet if you rest too much, your muscles can become weak and wasted (atrophied) from disuse, and your tendons and ligaments can even shorten and cause your joints to become deformed and incapable of straightening all the way. So although proper rest and sleep are important, proper exercise is just as important.

Exercise

Before the Twentieth Century, doctors thought that the best treatment for arthritis was rest. Now the experts believe that while rest may help in some situations, a proper balance between rest and exercise is more important. Exercise can combat many of the symptoms that can accompany arthritis, including fatigue, muscle atrophy, loss of stamina, stiffness, and even pain. It can also help prevent and can even correct some of the contractures that can develop in arthritis—the shortening of muscles, tendons, and ligaments that make it difficult or even impossible to straighten a joint completely. Exercise has a psychological benefit, too; faithful exercisers experience less stress, anxiety, and depression than those who don't exercise.

There are several different kinds of exercise that are beneficial to arthritis sufferers. Range of motion and stretching exercises are intended to keep the joints flexible so that you can use them easily. Muscle-strengthening exercises and aerobic exercises (the kind that speed up your heartbeat and make you breathe more deeply) build stamina and actually reduce fatigue, and they can even reduce pain. They are thought to do the latter by stimulating the release of endorphins, the body's own natural painkillers and tranquilizers, which are produced in the brain, the spinal cord, and the pituitary gland. To find an appropriate exercise regimen for yourself, you might look at a book like *Arthritis: Your Complete Exercise Guide,* by Neil F. Gordon, M.D., or you might visit an exercise center that caters to people with arthritis. The YMCA is one such place.

Exercise has its risks, though. Many forms of arthritis can also affect the heart and circulatory system (for example, rheumatoid arthritis and arthritis associated with systemic lupus erythematosus), and vigorous exercise can put a lot of stress on those tissues. And the wrong kind of exercise could further damage your joints. For example, for a person with moderate to severe osteoarthritis in the knees, a high-impact exercise like running may further damage the joint. Low-impact exercises, like walking, cycling, and swimming are preferable. In general, anyone wanting to start on an exercise program for arthritis should consult his or her doctor to find out what kind and level of exercise is best.

Heat

A long hot shower or bath can ease morning arthritis pain and stiffness. A heating pad or a thick, warm damp towel can work well, too, as long as you avoid burning yourself. Hydrotherapy—the swirling or pulsing warm water of a whirlpool bath, hot tub, or spa system—is also useful. Because the heat relaxes joints and muscles, it's a good idea to take a warm shower or bath before exercising.

Cold

For some people, cold may help, since it has a numbing effect. Gel-filled cold packs that can be kept in the freezer, or plastic bags full of ice chips can be applied to the painful area. But cold is dangerous, too—it can cause muscle spasms and circulatory disturbances, as well as frostbite, which can damage tissue that is kept too cold for too long.

Copper Bracelets

Copper is a trace mineral—that is, your body requires it, but only in tiny amounts. Copper bracelets are a folk remedy for aches and pains that dates back to ancient Greece. At one time such bracelets were looked upon as pure quackery. However, there is now evidence that people with rheumatoid arthritis have very low levels of copper in their bodies. Copper salts, which were investigated at the same time as gold salts, were shown to produce favorable results in people with rheumatic diseases. Unfortunately, they had too many bad side effects to be useful. But copper bracelets, which allow tiny amounts of copper to be absorbed through the skin, appear to work without those side effects. One study, cited in the exhaustive *Primer on the Rheumatic Diseases*, compared real copper bracelets to fake ones that looked the same (made of aluminum) and reported that arthritics wearing the real bracelets had less pain than the ones wearing the fakes. No negative side effects were reported.

Copper bracelets are not expensive, and they last for much longer than any human lifetime. On some people they may cause greenish or blackish stains where they touch the skin, due to the interaction of the copper with sweat and skin oil, but these stains (which actually contain tiny amounts of copper leached from the bracelet) wash off and are not harmful, although you may consider them unsightly.

Acupuncture

Acupuncture, a practice that has been part of Chinese medicine for the past two thousand years, consists of the insertion of fine stainless steel needles into the skin at certain places on the body in order to produce various effects. One of these intended effects is the relief of pain.

Traditional Chinese medicine holds that health is maintained by the balance of two opposing forces called *yin* and *yang*. When the two are unbalanced, a person becomes ill. The balance between yin and yang is controlled by an energy called *qi*, which flows along channels in our bodies. By appropriately altering the flow of qi, the proper balance between yin and yang can be restored. Along the channels are 361 places (called acupoints) where needles can be inserted to alter that flow. The application of heat or pressure (called acupressure) is also supposed to be able to do the job.

There is evidence that acupuncture works fairly well, not just for pain but for drug addiction, some types of nausea, and some nerve disorders. Researchers have found that many acupoints lie over or close to places where major nerves meet muscle or bone; stimulation of such places may account for acupuncture's ability to alleviate pain. Other researchers have found evidence that acupuncture promotes the release of endorphins, the body's own natural, internal painkillers. However it works, acupuncture appears to be able to benefit 55 to 85 percent of patients with chronic pain.

Acupuncture does carry some risk. With needles being stuck into your skin, there is risk of infection or even transmission of blood-borne diseases, like AIDS. Because of this, most practitioners now use one-time-only disposable needles. You should, of course, check to make sure your acupuncturist uses these.

A single acupuncture treatment may help your arthritis pain, but it's more likely that you would need four to twenty treatments (at two or three treatments a week) to get significant relief. How long such relief would last is not known. This can get expensive. Acupuncture can cost ninety-five dollars or more for the first treatment, and seventy-five dollars or more for each follow-up, and your insurance may not cover it. (For example, in Illinois, State Farm Insurance and Blue Cross-Blue Shield don't cover acupuncture.)

SURGERY

Surgery is the last resort when arthritic joints are so damaged or so painful that nothing else does any good. There are two types of surgery used to treat arthritis, arthroscopic and arthroplastic.

In arthroscopic surgery, a tiny camera and instruments inserted through small incisions allow the surgeon to remove bone fragments and damaged cartilage.

In arthroplasty, the joint itself is removed and replaced by an artificial joint made of metal and plastic. The hip, knee, shoulder, elbow, finger, wrist, and ankle joints can all be replaced. Although the artificial joint doesn't work as well as a natural one would, it usually works better than the old one did, and most people are happy with their new joint. The major drawback to joint replacement is that the joint is attached to the remaining bone by pins and cement, which can wear, loosen, and break and can't repair themselves as real bone and tissue could. The replacement joint will only last a limited period of time, and therefore the surgery will eventually have to be repeated, perhaps fifteen or twenty years down the line. For that reason, some doctors are reluctant to perform this surgery on a relatively young person. But most people who turn to joint replacement are willing to accept the possibility that it will have to be re-done in the future.

The greatest risk in joint replacement is infection, which can make the artificial joint loosen and fail, forcing its removal. Treating such infections is very difficult.

Are there any other options? Is there anything that is non-invasive, without unpleasant and even life-threatening side effects, and easy to use? Anything that won't require endless visits to some specialist or long periods of recovery? Anything that won't involve being stuck or cut or put in a plaster cast? Anything else that a person with arthritis can try, that has worked on other people?

Yes! Pantothenic acid. And in the next chapter we'll tell you exactly what that is.

Chapter 4

WHAT IS PANTOTHENIC ACID?

Unless you are in the habit of reading the labels on multivitamin bottles, you have probably never heard of pantothenic acid. Yet, every day of your life, this substance flows through your bloodstream, reaching every organ of your body. In this chapter, we'll take a look at what it is and why we need it so much.

WHAT ARE VITAMINS?

Vitamins are complex substances, made mainly of carbon, hydrogen, oxygen, and nitrogen, that our bodies need to stay alive. Vitamins do not provide energy themselves, but they enable us to transform the food we eat into energy. They are not part of any of the structures of the human body—the bones, the muscles, the nerves—but they allow us to build those structures and maintain them. Every time we walk to the corner drug store for a newspaper or carry a load of laundry to the washing machine, we are drawing on the activity of vitamins; every time we get out of bed in the morning, vitamins have made it possible. Without enough vitamins, children cannot grow properly; without enough vitamins, adults and children can suffer dangerous deficiency diseases. Without any vitamins at all, our bodies would simply stop functioning.

Fortunately, vitamins occur in the foods we eat, so we take them in at every meal. There they are, right in the middle of all that raw material of proteins, fats, starches, and sugars. And their job is to help that raw material through the process of breakdown and buildup, of energy production and use, that is called *metabolism*. Vitamins move in and out of the various chemical reactions of metabolism in much the same way a bricklayer builds a wall; the bricklayer moves the bricks around, and he may even dip his hands into the mortar, but at the end of the day, he leaves the wall to stand on its own and goes home for dinner. At the end of the process of metabolism, the vitamins have done their jobs, but they have not been consumed—they have not been turned into energy or body structures. They have either been stored in the body for future use, or they have been flushed out and will need to be replaced very soon.

Whether vitamins are stored or flushed out depends, in general, on whether they are oil-soluble or water-soluble. These are the two grand classes of vitamins. The oil-soluble vitamins, A, D, E, and K, can be stored in the body's liver or fatty tissues for many months. Once taken in, they are ready to be used whenever raw materials present themselves, even if that particular meal doesn't contain much A, D, E, or K. Because of this long-term storage, it is relatively easy to overdose on them by taking large supplements for any extended period of time—the kinds of large supplements available in single-vitamin capsules at drug or health food stores.

Water-soluble vitamins, on the other hand, are stored for very short periods of time. They are readily flushed out of the body in urine and must be frequently replaced. This flushing process is easy to observe in the case of one member of the B complex family of vitamins: riboflavin (vitamin B_2). Riboflavin is bright yellow in color, and a few hours after you swallow a capsule or tablet containing a large amount of it, your urine takes on that unmistakable color, as a large proportion of the vitamin is eliminated from your body. Some people believe this is a sign that this large amount of riboflavin is being wasted. In reality, all of the riboflavin consumed even in the usual way (in food) is flushed out of the body unchanged and fairly quickly, whether it has been used in aiding metabolism or not; the amount in one typical day's meals is just never enough to color urine perceptibly.

The other water soluble vitamins include vitamin C and the rest of the B complex: thiamine (vitamin B_1), niacin (vitamin B_3), pantothenic acid (vitamin B_5), pyridoxine (vitamin B_6), cyanocobalamine (vitamin B_{12}), folic acid, and biotin. Some of these vitamins are familiar to most people. Who hasn't heard of vitamin C, found in orange juice and added to beverages as diverse as cranberry juice cocktail, Hawaiian Punch, and Tang? Some of the B vitamins should be nearly as familiar to anyone who reads cereal boxes or bread wrappers. These foods are routinely enriched with thiamine, riboflavin, and niacin, as well as with iron. Folic acid (also known as folate) is the newest candidate for public awareness, in its role as a substance that, when taken by pregnant women, appears to prevent certain birth defects in their babies, especially spina bifida. Folic acid has lately joined the list of vitamins added to cereals ranging from Kellogg's Raisin Bran to General Mills' Count Chocula.

Probably least known of the B vitamins is pantothenic acid. Every multivitamin tablet contains some. As a stand-alone vitamin, it's on the shelf at most drugstores that stock individual vitamins, usually near the niacin. *The Encyclopedia Britannica* has an article on it. But most doctors find its name unfamiliar. The people who know the most about it tend to be biochemists, and even they know it by another name (see The Master Enzyme later in this chapter).

The Discovery of Pantothenic Acid

The 1920s and 30s were the heyday of vitamin research. Thiamine, the first vitamin to be discovered, was isolated in pure form in 1926 and synthesized in 1936. Vitamin A's chemical structure was determined in 1933. Riboflavin, niacin, vitamin B_6, vitamin C, folic acid, biotin, vitamin D, vitamin E, and vitamin K were all discovered, recognized, or synthesized during this period. The history of pantothenic acid is the typically collaborative story of the unmasking of a vitamin.

If pantothenic acid had a single discoverer, that person was Roger J. Williams, who, for nearly forty years, was a professor of chemistry at the University of Texas at Austin. In 1933 he published the first scientific article identifying a substance that was water soluble and acidic, and stimulated growth in yeast. It was present in extracts from many different plant and animal tissues, and because of that, he coined the name "pantothenic acid" for it, from the Greek word "pantos," meaning "everywhere." He had isolated it from yeast in crystalline form, and he thought it was a vitamin.

Researchers were investigating deficiency diseases quite a lot in those days, trying to determine what substances were lacking in the diets of people with ailments like rickets, beriberi, and pellagra, and what could be added to those diets to cure them. Most of this research was done on animals, of course, and one of the deficiency diseases that cropped up among the baby chicks often used for these experiments was something called "chick dermatitis."

Chick dermatitis may sound fairly trivial, but it isn't. Human dermatitis is an inflammation of the skin accompanied by itching; dandruff is one variety (seborrheic dermatitis)—annoying, but not life threatening. Chick dermatitis, however, is just a shorthand name for a whole array of symptoms. Dermatitis refers to the crusty scabs that occur at the corners of a chick's mouth, which enlarge over time and spread to all the skin around the base of the beak. It also includes the thickening of the skin of the chick's feet, where small cracks soon appear, enlarging and deepening steadily, and sometimes bleeding. Chicks with feet like these walk gingerly, obviously in pain. They have trouble with their eyes, too, the edges of the lids becoming granular and exuding a gummy substance, often sticking together so completely that the chicks can't see. Their feathers come in later than usual, and those that finally emerge are rough and stand out, bristling, rather than lying smooth against their bodies, as a bird's feathers should. Internally, the chicks show serious liver and spinal cord damage. And, overall, chicks with dermatitis are smaller than healthy ones.

To induce this syndrome, researchers purposely fed chicks certain kinds of very limited diets, known to include some vital nutrients, but thought to be lacking in others not yet identified. That must have been true, because by the end of one twelve-week study, half the chicks were dead.

Chick dermatitis was clearly a deficiency disease, but a deficiency of what? What nutrient, left out or destroyed in the preparation of these diets, would cure it? In 1930, scientists added yeast to a limited chick diet, and the chicks recovered completely and resumed normal growth. Something was in the yeast that counteracted the deficiency. But yeast contains many different nutrients. Which one was it? As purified and synthesized vitamins became available, they were tested on chick dermatitis. Riboflavin didn't work; that was tried in 1935. Niacin didn't work; that was 1938. Thiamine and B_6 were failures, too. There had to be something else vital to healthy chick life in the yeast.

One substance did work, though it had nothing to do

with yeast. Liver extract from which the riboflavin and all its close relatives (the other flavins) had been removed cured chick dermatitis nicely. Since the flavins were removed by filtering the extract through fuller's earth (a fine-grained, clay-like material), the unknown substance was dubbed "filtrate factor" by some experimenters. Others preferred to call it "chick anti-dermatitis factor" because, after all, that was exactly what it was. In 1939, two sets of independent researchers finally pointed out that the chemical properties of filtrate factor (alias chick anti-dermatitis factor) were just like the chemical properties of Williams' pantothenic acid. Testing on chicks followed and proved the case. Williams had been right: pantothenic acid cured a deficiency disease; it was a vitamin, at least for chicks.

Investigating the Deficiency

In 1940, Williams and a colleague synthesized pure pantothenic acid, which, by eliminating the possibility of contaminants, made investigating its properties much simpler. Subsequently, the focus of most of the research on pantothenic acid moved away from chicks. The reason for this is simple: although chicks are readily available (and investigators in all realms of science, from biology to psychology, still use them), they are not the best possible models for vitamin use in the creatures we are all most interested in—human beings. They are not, after all, mammals. The mammals most commonly used in scientific research are, like chicks, small and easy to handle and care for. They mature quickly and reproduce in large numbers. And, like human beings, they'll eat pretty much anything. They are, of course, rats.

We are all most familiar with white rats, but laboratory rats come in a variety of coat colors. And it was a change in coat color that was one of the first symptoms of pantothenic acid deficiency noticed in these animals. In 1938, researchers reported that after eight to twelve weeks on a diet deficient in filtrate factor (it hadn't been identified as pantothenic acid yet), the fur of black and brown rats began to turn gray. Rats fed exactly the same diet with filtrate factor retained their normal fur color. And when the graying rats were given filtrate factor, the new fur that grew in had their old dark color.

During the next twenty years of research into this deficiency, other, far more serious symptoms were observed, and the same ones were reported over and over again. Sometimes these symptoms took months to appear, a long time in the short life of a rat, but they did appear. Dermatitis was one of them—a sloughing of spots and patches of skin that led to ulcerations that would not heal. Patches of fur would fall out, the rats would have nosebleeds, and their eyes would exude gummy matter. An adult rat would lose weight on the pantothenic acid deficient diet, a young rat would grow abnormally slowly and never reach the normal size of its non-deprived littermates. If a female rat were put on the diet from the day of mating, her offspring would never live to the age of weaning (twenty-one days). If she were put on it the day her offspring were born, and if they continued on it after weaning, they rarely survived past forty days. Those that survived the longest showed the same symptoms as pantothenic acid deficient adults. Sudden and unexpected death of the experimental animals, no matter how old they were, was the rule in these deprivation studies.

Autopsies of the rats showed what the deficiency had done to them internally. In reporting on the results of the autopsies, researchers frequently used the word "necrotic"; it means "the dying of a part of the body while the rest is still alive." Obviously, a necrotic organ is not going to function the way it is supposed to. Two of the rats' most important organs were necrotic: the kidneys and the adrenal glands. In addition, the rats' hearts had enlarged or hemorrhaged, the rats had intestinal ulcers, and if they were young when the deficiency period started, their bone growth was badly retarded and their bone marrow abnormal.

In the 1950s, scientists determined that a pantothenic acid deficiency also lowered the rats' resistance to infection (a large proportion of them died of pneumonia) by impairing their ability to make antibodies. Pantothenic acid was indeed necessary for rat life.

Inevitably, research was performed on other kinds of animals—guinea pigs, calves, pigs, and dogs. Eventually, several things became clear from all these animal studies.

First, pantothenic acid deficiency did produce life-threatening symptoms in mammals, symptoms that affected some of the most important tissues of the body—the adrenal glands, the kidneys, the heart, the digestive system, the bones.

Second, except in animals who nursed with deficient mothers, the external symptoms were slow to appear, taking as long as five to seven weeks to become obvious.

Third, the symptoms could be reversed, and the animal's health and life saved, if supplements of pantothenic acid were given in time.

Still, these were all animal studies. How much like human beings are chicks, rats, dogs, calves, pigs, and guinea pigs? There are important differences. For example, every one of these animals, except the guinea pig, never suffers from vitamin C deficiency (scurvy); they can all synthesize vitamin C in their own bodies. But guinea pigs, human beings, and our primate relatives must acquire vitamin C from outside sources. (That's one of the major reasons why guinea pigs became the proverbial experimental animal, although their use has limitations because they are strict vegetarians, unlike most human beings.)

Somebody had to do human studies. But human studies require volunteers, and who would volunteer, knowing that the research was potentially life-threatening?

The Deficiency in Human Beings

Beriberi is a deficiency disease caused by a lack of thiamine, pellagra is caused by a lack of niacin, and scurvy is caused by a lack of vitamin C. Each of them is cured by adding the missing vitamin to the sufferer's diet. But the diseases themselves were known and named long before the vitamins that cure them were identified. Pantothenic acid deficiency does not have a common name because it has so rarely been observed in human beings, or at least so rarely recognized. Most of its outward symptoms also occur in other deficiency diseases, which makes distinguishing it from others very difficult. Other deficiency diseases may well mask a pantothenic acid deficiency. In 1940, a researcher discovered that patients with pellagra, beriberi, or riboflavin deficiency also had 25 to 50 percent less pantothenic acid in their blood than normal people.

Because pantothenic acid occurs in so many different animal and plant tissues, anyone who eats a reasonably varied diet takes in some of it. But there are circumstances where that isn't possible. There is a disease, known since 1826, called "nutritional melalgia" or "burning feet syndrome." In it, not only do the feet burn, but aches and pains shoot up the legs. It occurs in people with severe malnutrition, the kind of malnutrition that can happen in wartime. During World War II, prisoners of war in Japan and the Philippines, living on extremely limited diets, suffered from burning feet syndrome, and this was the only symptom they exhibited that could not be attributed to a deficiency of some other vitamin. Shortly after the war, a doctor in India reported on some patients with this syndrome who did not respond to either niacin or thiamine (thiamine actually made them worse) but were cured with pantothenic acid.

That was all that was known about pantothenic acid deficiency in human beings up to the early 1950s. Then, two investigators at the University of Iowa in Iowa City decided to study the effects of pantothenic acid deficiency in healthy young human beings. They needed volunteers who would be willing to spend all of their time for at least ten weeks in a controlled environment (the Metabolic Ward of the Department of Internal Medicine at the University's medical school) where everything they consumed could be monitored. They found their volunteers about thirty-five miles away, at the Anamosa State Reformatory: four healthy men ranging in age from nineteen to thirty-one.

At the very beginning of the study there were problems. Information existed on the amounts of pantothenic acid found in various foods, but when it was double-checked, most of it turned out to be wrong. So instead of using ordinary foods in measured amounts, the researchers decided to concoct a purified and mostly synthetic diet with every known vitamin and important mineral added to it, except pantothenic acid. And because their goal was to make sure the volunteers were completely deficient in pantothenic acid, they would give the men one of the newly-discovered pantothenic acid antagonists, which would block the action of any of the vitamin that might somehow manage to sneak into their special diet.

Today, because of tighter ethical guidelines developed by scientists, such an experiment would not be allowed. It would be considered too dangerous for human beings. But forty years ago, attitudes—at least among some researchers—were different.

The first twelve days of the study were the baseline period, with the volunteers consuming the special diet, plus some pantothenic acid, but not the antagonist. In its nutritional levels, this diet mimicked an ordinary, healthy level of eating. During this baseline time, and for the rest of the study, thirty aspects of the men's health were recorded regularly, including weight, blood pressure, appetite, general sense of well-being, and the results of various blood and urine tests. The men felt fine for the baseline period, and their health looked normal. Then the pantothenic acid was discontinued and the antagonist begun.

The second period of the study, the time they were on the deficient and antagonist diet, lasted seven weeks. During this time, their earliest symptoms included disturbances of blood pressure, feelings of vertigo, abnormally fast heart rates after only slight exertion, upper abdominal pains, constipation, and loss of appetite. Other symptoms included easy irritability and fatigue. The subjects tired quickly and often slept during the daytime. Later symptoms included sensations of numbness and tingling in the hands and feet. One subject's feet burned constantly for the last three weeks of the period, another developed an odd way of walking, like a goose-step, and another was plagued by itching and prickling much of the time. They had various muscular weaknesses and an impaired sense of balance. A few of their blood tests were abnormal. And for the whole seven weeks they all had frequent respiratory infections; one of them even came down with pneumonia.

In the third period of the study, the subjects continued the diet of the second period, but with massive doses of pantothenic acid added. These were intended to overwhelm the antagonist and return the men to normal health. Unfortunately, the massive doses didn't work, or at least they didn't work soon enough. Over the course of the next six days, the fatigue became worse. In one case a subject was drowsy for an entire day; another subject started vomiting. At that point the investigators finally decided that their subjects were showing signs of acute adrenal insufficiency—a lack of the hormones normally secreted by the adrenal gland. Because adrenal insufficiency can lead to sudden death, the researchers terminated the study and gave the men emergency therapy: intravenous fluids, cortisone (one of the adrenal hormones), real food, and large vitamin supplements, including pantothenic acid. It took the men more than three weeks to recover from their ordeal.

Over the period of deficiency, the subjects had lost weight steadily, even though they had consumed 3,000 calories a day, an amount that should have easily maintained (or even increased) their initial weights, especially considering the limited exercise they got while living in the Metabolic Ward. (These days the typical healthy adult diet is assumed to be 2,000-2,500 calories, according to the government-mandated labeling you can find on almost any food container.) The researchers made nothing of this interesting fact, but we will come back to it later in this chapter.

As far as the researchers could tell, the subjects of this study recovered their health completely, although there was no long-term follow-up on them once they appeared to be back to normal. The subjects were not autopsied, of course (since they weren't dead), and many tests now available, like the CAT scan or the MRI, did not exist in the 1950s, so it was impossible to determine if any of their organs were necrotic. But those symptoms of adrenal insufficiency were suspicious, and the abnormal blood and urine tests pointed at lowered adrenal activity as well.

Having learned a few things from this study, the same investigators recruited a third scientist to help them with a another, more elaborate study of pantothenic acid deficiency, using six fresh volunteers from the Reformatory. The results were pretty much the same, except that diarrhea was added to the list of symptoms, and the volunteers didn't get quite so dangerously ill this time (or perhaps the investigators just didn't panic when the men didn't feel up to getting out of bed all day). But toward the end of the study, their coordination—as measured by their ability to play Ping-Pong at the end of the study compared to the baseline period—had deteriorated badly, and when they walked, they staggered.

In both studies, the researchers noted that the men did not react identically to pantothenic acid deficiency. They varied in how long the symptoms took to appear, in exactly which symptoms were exhibited by each, and how bad they were. This had been true of the rats, too. The researchers attributed these differences to natural individual variability. We all know about this variability, of course—it's the reason why some people catch colds and others don't, why some are allergic to wool, or feathers, or ragweed, or penicillin, and others are not. Variability permeates our lives, and it's a topic we'll return to in a later chapter.

Other scientists followed up on this work with another human study in 1976, and again got much the same results. Pantothenic acid was definitely necessary for human well-being, as well as for other animals.

Yet in all of this research, the full-blown deficiency took weeks to show up, suggesting that in spite of being water-soluble and readily lost in the urine, some amount of pantothenic acid was being stored in the body—be it rat, calf, or human—for long periods of time.

Human studies of excretion of pantothenic acid in the urine supported that suggestion. At high intakes of the vitamin, or even at modest intakes, substantial amounts of pantothenic acid were not excreted, but were retained by the body. When people who had previously consumed large amounts of the vitamin were switched to a low pantothenic acid diet, they actually began to excrete more of the vitamin than they took in, and this continued for at least fifteen days (the duration of that experiment). They had obviously stored quite a bit during the high-intake period. On the other hand, people who had been kept on a low pantothenic acid diet for forty-two days did not show an increase in their excretion when the amount of the vitamin in their diet was increased, as if they were replenishing their bodies' depleted stores from the new, larger supply.

When the second group of volunteers from the Reformatory were on pantothenic acid deficient diets, their excretion of the vitamin fell quickly to nearly zero, but when they were given massive doses of the vitamin daily for two weeks after their period of deficiency, they excreted only one-quarter of it each following day. This was a small amount compared to what they were taking in, but much more than would be excreted by the average person eating an ordinary diet. The study ended two weeks after these extra-large doses had been discontinued and the men had returned to ordinary diets, but their excretion levels were still well above normal at that point. The body obviously gets rid of extra pantothenic acid pretty slowly.

What is this substance? It is extremely important—we know that from all these studies. But what, exactly, does it do?

THE MASTER ENZYME

Our bodies stay alive and healthy because of the myriad of chemical reactions that make up the metabolism. We take in food made of proteins, carbohydrates (sugars and starches), and fats. The complex chemical factory that is the human body breaks that food up, builds new substances out of some of it, turns some of it into energy, stores some of it for future use, and gets rid of the rest through urine, feces, sweat, and the breath we exhale. That process begins the moment we put food in our mouths, and it continues as the food is chewed and swallowed and moves through the stomach and intestines. All along the way, substances called *enzymes* work on the food, gradually breaking it down into simpler and simpler pieces, and in the intestine it undergoes the final fragmenting that will allow it to be absorbed by the intestinal walls and passed to other parts of the body for the next stage of processing.

Vitamins are not broken down by this process because they are ready to be used as they are. They pass through the intestinal walls unchanged. Pantothenic acid, like the other water-soluble vitamins, then enters the bloodstream and circulates with the blood throughout the body. When it reaches an organ, like the heart, the adrenal glands, or the liver, or when it just attaches itself to a red blood cell, it temporarily picks up two chemical appendages that hook on to either end of the vitamin. In this form, it is known as coenzyme A.

An enzyme is a substance that either makes a chemical reaction run or makes it run faster, and at the end of that reaction, the enzyme is still there in its original form. Nature (and the food we eat) is full of enzymes; some we even make ourselves, building them inside our bodies from smaller parts. Without enzymes, life would be impossible, and more than a thousand of them have been identified so far.

If an enzyme doesn't work properly, disease can happen. For example, people with phenylketonuria can't make an active form of the enzyme needed to process the amino acid phenylalanine (amino acids are fragments of protein). Yet many foods contain phenylalanine, and so as these foods are eaten, the phenylalanine builds up and builds up in tissues, its abnormal presence interfering with normal metabolism. The domino effect of one interrupted reaction preventing the occurrence of another that depends on it eventually results in nerve damage, mental retardation, and seizures. The only way to avoid the damage is to eat a special diet that contains no phenylalanine, which is why foods and beverages sweetened with the artificial sweetener aspartame, which contains phenylalanine, have a warning to phenylketonurics on their labels.

If an enzyme is merely not in adequate supply rather than inactive, the chemical reactions that depend on it don't occur as frequently as they should. There is a domino effect here, too, because so many of the body's functions are interdependent. Too little of one enzyme can cause a whole series of chemical reactions to move at a crawl rather than a gallop; all sorts of substances that the body needs end up in short supply; processes that are necessary to health and life can't be maintained at their proper levels. The living creature that is the sum of all these parts deteriorates.

Some enzymes are made of two sections that link up with each other in the body, and both parts are necessary for the enzyme to do its job. One variety of such a composite enzyme has a protein section, called an apoenzyme, and a section made from a vitamin, called a coenzyme. Niacin, biotin, vitamin B_6, and pantothenic acid can all form coenzymes. And coenzyme A, made from pantothenic acid, is the most important of them all.

No one really understood the significance of pantothenic acid in human (or any other) metabolism until coenzyme A was discovered in 1947. Since that time, its crucial importance to a host of metabolic processes has been intensively studied. Even so, pantothenic acid itself is not nearly as well-known as the famous coenzyme A. It's just the center section, the indispensable heart, of that substance. Say "pantothenic acid" to a biochemist and he might well shrug and shake his head; the name doesn't sound familiar. Say "coenzyme A," and he knows exactly what that means.

In the simplest terms, coenzyme A takes small pieces of chemical substances and moves them from one place to another. In the jargon of biochemistry, it is an *acyl carrier*. This modest title cloaks a very large responsibility.

First and foremost, coenzyme A is at the hub of the set of reactions known as the TCA cycle (tricarboxylic acid cycle), which uses proteins, carbohydrates, and fats to produce two-thirds of the energy that all the cells of our bodies need to function. That is two-thirds of all the energy that powers our life processes, from the muscle contractions that allow us to walk to the nerve transmissions that allow us to think. If this cycle fails, there is another way to produce energy, but it isn't nearly as efficient; it doesn't produce the quantities of energy that our bodies truly need. Without coenzyme A, the TCA cycle comes to a dead stop.

Second, but hardly less important, coenzyme A helps to manufacture a wide variety of specific substances that our bodies use, including acetylcholine and the steroid hormones testosterone, progesterone, aldosterone, and cortisol. Acetylcholine is one of the chemicals that transmits signals from one nerve to another. Testosterone is the sex hormone responsible for the development of masculine characteristics. Progesterone acts on the female organs, its main job being to prepare the lining of the uterus for implantation of a fertilized egg. Aldosterone, made in the adrenal glands, regulates sodium, potassium, and water balance in the body. Cortisol, also made in the adrenal glands (and readily transformed into its close relative, cortisone), primarily helps to control sugar levels in the blood and liver, although it also affects many other parts of the body, including the central nervous system, the lymph nodes, the intestines, and the connective tissues (bones, ligaments, tendons, cartilage, skin, and fatty tissue). Coenzyme A itself also helps to manufacture some important components of that connective tissue. In all of these manufacturing processes, nothing else can take the place of coenzyme A.

Coenzyme A is found in every part of the body, and in the largest concentrations in the internal organs—the heart, liver, kidneys, adrenal glands, and brain. The liver, the central factory of the body, has the highest concentration, followed by the adrenal glands. Scientists think that whatever amounts of pantothenic acid are stored by the body can be found in these internal organs in the form of coenzyme A. Amounts that are not stored are stripped back to plain pantothenic acid, returned to the blood and, if not re-used, then flushed out in the urine.

We can now guess at the reasons for some of the deficiency symptoms both animals and humans experience, especially the early ones that set in well before the interference with so many bodily processes becomes great enough to cause death. A lowered level of energy production would surely lead to general tiredness and a loss of the sense of well-being. If the adrenal glands could not make their hormones, they might well become damaged; certainly if they aren't making those hormones, that situation is exactly "adrenal insufficiency." Nervous system problems like poor coordination (poor performance at Ping-Pong) could be caused by a deficit of acetylcholine.

Other symptoms, such as weight loss, lack of weight gain in spite of large food intake, and digestive disorders like diarrhea may be the result of an inability to process food properly because the systems that are supposed to process it don't have enough energy to do so—the sagging TCA cycle.

But this is all theoretical, isn't it? Pantothenic acid is so widespread in the modern diet, at least in America, that nobody outside a scientific study is pantothenic acid deficient these days. Right?

The answer is, maybe not, as we'll see in the next chapter.

Chapter 5

DO WE GET ENOUGH PANTOTHENIC ACID?

For years, the accepted wisdom of medical science and of the U.S. Food and Drug Administration has been that anyone who eats a well-balanced diet gets all the vitamins he or she needs from food. Therefore, supplements are not only not necessary, they are a waste of money. Yet some 40 percent of American adults take vitamin supplements. Are they wrong? Or is the FDA?

Since our focus is on pantothenic acid, in this chapter we'll look at that supposed well-balanced diet and find out if it really does contain all of the pantothenic acid that we should be getting.

THE DAILY VALUE

According to the FDA, the Daily Values of the vitamins (known until recently as the Recommended Daily Allowances or RDA) represent the highest amounts of those vitamins that are needed by most people each day. These are the amounts that will not only stave off deficiency diseases like beriberi, pellagra, and scurvy, but will maintain the human body in a healthy state, assuming that appropriate quantities of the raw materials that vitamins work with (proteins, carbohydrates, and fats) are also consumed.

Amounts of the water-soluble vitamins, including pantothenic acid, are measured by weight, using the metric system. A gram (abbreviated "g") is the basic unit of weight, and 28.3 grams equals one ounce. A milligram ("mg") is one thousandth of a gram. As you'll see by reading the label on any multivitamin bottle, the Daily Value for pantothenic acid is 10 mg.

SOURCES OF PANTOTHENIC ACID

Pantothenic acid's name comes from a Greek word ("pantos") meaning "everywhere," and the vitamin is indeed found in most foods, but only in small amounts. Among non-meats, mushrooms are by far the most abundant natural source of pantothenic acid, but you would have to eat a pound of raw mushrooms to take in the Daily Value. The next highest (non-meat) natural source is broccoli, and you would have to eat nearly two pounds of raw broccoli to achieve the Daily Value. Other vegetables are even lower in pantothenic acid. Fruits and fruit juices are lower still.

Among meats, liver has the most pantothenic acid by far; you would only have to eat about four and a half ounces of broiled fresh liver to get the Daily Value. Fresh chicken, beef, pork, and fish (all either broiled or baked) have substantially less pantothenic acid than liver, though they are all better sources than most vegetables. (See Table 5.1 for good sources of pantothenic acid.)

You'll notice the words "raw" and "fresh" above. The reason for their use is that once you cook, can, or freeze food, its

Food Source	Pantothenic Acid (mg)
Meats	
chuck steak (3 oz)	.72
lean ground beef (3 oz)	.63
chicken (3 oz)	1.01
loin pork chop (3 oz)	.55
liver (beef, pork, lamb) (3 oz)	6.54
kidneys (beef, pork, lamb) (3 oz)	3.82
beef brains (3 oz)	1.53
beef heart (3 oz)	1.76
liverwurst (3 oz)	1.90
salami (3 oz)	.85
Dairy and eggs	
1 egg (2 oz)	.62
1 cup skim milk	.80
Fish	
salmon (3 oz)	1.10
Grains	
1 cup cooked brown rice (6 oz)	.60
1/2 cup (measured dry) oatmeal	.60
Vegetables	
1 medium tomato (7 oz)	.65
1 cup broccoli (3 oz)	.99
1 cup cauliflower (3 oz)	.85
1 cup kale (3 oz)	.85
1 cup mushrooms (2 oz)	1.24
1 medium sweet potato (6.4 oz)	1.48

If cooked, meat and fish are broiled or baked without added water. Vegetables are raw, except for sweet potato, which is baked in its skin. (Sources: Schroeder 1977; Walsh 1981; Marks 1975; Novelli 1953; Carnation powdered milk label 1995.)

Table 5.1 Some Foods High in Pantothenic Acid.

vitamin content, and its pantothenic acid content in particular, falls. We'll take another look at this crucial aspect of nutrition after we examine the concept of the well-balanced diet. After all, most people don't normally eat—and wouldn't really want to eat—two pounds of broccoli a day, or a pound of mushrooms, either raw or cooked. And they probably wouldn't want to eat four and a half ounces of liver that often, either. Most people like the idea of eating a varied diet, and that's where the Food Pyramid comes in.

THE WELL-BALANCED DIET

The Food Pyramid (seen so frequently on bread wrappers and cracker boxes these days) and the new government-mandated "Nutrition Facts" labeling on most food packages are supposed to be our guides to proper nutrition through a well-balanced diet. The Pyramid, shown in Figure 5.1, divides foods into six categories and tells how many servings from each category should be included for a healthy total intake of food in one day.

Each chart of Nutrition Facts lists the size of one serving of the food in that particular package and how much nutrition it contains, in terms of the Daily Value. Table 5.2 shows a typical Nutrition Facts chart, in this case from the label on a loaf of a leading brand of natural wheat bread. You'll notice that there are official Daily Values for fat, cholesterol, sodium, carbohydrates, and fiber, as well as for vitamins A and C and the minerals calcium and iron; the chart gives the bread's percentages of all of them.

To explain the concept of "Daily Value," the label also includes the information in Table 5.3, which notes that the Daily Values are based on a 2,000 calorie diet. (This implies, of course, that 2,000 calories a day is an appropriate number of calories for the average American adult, and many authorities agree with that, considering how little exercise most of

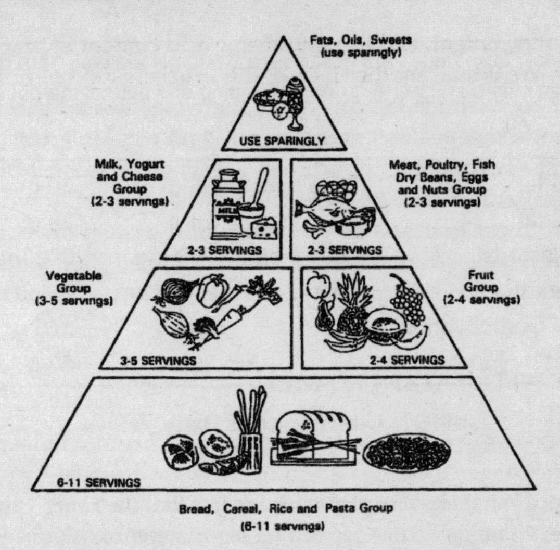

Figure 5.1 The Food Guide Pyramid.

Serving size: 1 slice (36g) Servings per container: 19

Amount Per Serving

Calories 80		Calories from fat 10	
	% Daily Value*		% Daily Value*
Total Fat 1g	2%	**Total Carbohydrate** 17g	6%
Saturated Fat 0g	0%	Dietary Fiber 2g	8%
Cholesterol 0 mg	0%	Sugars less than 1g	
Sodium 200 mg	8%	**Protein** 3g	

Vitamin A 0% Vitamin C 0% Calcium 0% Iron 4%

*Percent Daily Values are based on a 2,000 calorie diet. Your daily values may be higher or lower depending on your calorie needs.

Table 5.2 Nutrition Facts From Label of a Leading Brand of Natural Wheat Bread.

Percent Daily Values are based on a 2,000 calorie diet. Your daily values may be higher or lower depending on your calorie needs:

	Calories:	2,000	2,500
Total fat	Less than	65 g	80 g
Sat fat	Less than	20 g	25 g
Cholesterol	Less than	300 mg	300 mg
Sodium	Less than	2,400 mg	2,400 mg
Total Carbohydrate		300 g	375 g
Dietary Fiber		25 g	30 g

Table 5.3 Explanation of Daily Values.

us get.) What is not explained is the fact that the Daily Values of the vitamins do not depend on the number of calories you take in. The Daily Value of vitamin C, for example, is 60 mg, no matter how many calories you consume. If a slice of this bread contained any vitamin C, that amount would be a percentage of 60 mg.

To complete its nutritional information, this label, like many others, also has a list of ingredients:

> Ground whole wheat, water, unbleached enriched flour [flour, malted barley, niacin, reduced iron, thiamine mononitrate, (vitamin B_1) and riboflavin (vitamin B_2)], high fructose corn syrup, partially hydrogenated soybean oil, salt, yeast, vinegar.

Now, if we put all this information together, we can come to some conclusions about the nutritional value of a slice of this natural wheat bread. We can see, for example, that it is one serving from the food group we should be eating the most of (bread, cereal, rice, pasta). If we ate six slices, we would be within the Pyramid's suggested range for number of servings per day. Six slices would also give us 480 calories, with only 12 percent of the 2,000 calorie diet's suggested level of fat. They would also provide 48 percent of our fiber quota for the day, and 24 percent of our iron. On all these counts, this bread looks like pretty healthy stuff. On the down side, though, our slices don't contain any vitamin A or vitamin C at all, so those would have to come from somewhere else. But since we have 1,520 calories left to play with, out of the recommended 2,000 per day, we can feel free to put something on those bread slices to supply that missing nutrition.

The bread also contains the B vitamins niacin, B_1, and B_2, but we can't tell how much because the labeling requirements don't call for that information. We don't know if the bread contains any pantothenic acid; pantothenic acid isn't mentioned anywhere on this label. In fact, you won't find pantothenic acid mentioned on the vast majority of labels at the supermarket. Well, why should it be? Indeed, why should any of those B vitamins be mentioned on those labels?

ENRICHING OUR FOOD

White flour, the kind you buy in five-pound bags at the supermarket, the kind that most breads and cookies and pasta are made of, is a highly processed foodstuff. Wheat, as it comes from the farmer's field, is full of vitamins, but by the time that wheat has been milled into white flour, much of its vitamin content is gone, removed with all the substances that give natural wheat its darker color—the bran and the germ. The same is true of white rice, which starts out with a vitamin-rich brown outer coating of bran that is removed in milling. White flour and white rice are "enriched" by adding back in some of the vitamins that have been removed during processing. But pantothenic acid is not added back in.

Ready-to-eat breakfast cereals are highly processed too, and many of them are also enriched with added vitamins, to replace the ones that have been stripped away, or even to increase the nutritional value of the cereal beyond its original, unprocessed content. Listed with the other ingredients on the cereal package, these vitamins typically include B_1, B_2, niacin (or its equivalent cousin, niacinamide), B_6, and B_{12}, though sometimes C and D are also added. Lately, some cereals have added another B vitamin, folic acid (also called folacin), because recent research indicates that supplements of this vitamin taken by women before and during pregnancy can prevent spina bifida and cleft palate in their babies.

A survey of seventy-seven cereals found on supermarket shelves reveals that only seven of them list pantothenic acid (as calcium pantothenate, an equivalent form) among their added vitamins.

Of eight breakfast bars, only one listed pantothenic acid; of eight pancake mixes, only two listed it. Even a well-known, vitamin-rich milk flavoring only adds pantothenic acid to one of its three flavors!

At the supermarket, you can find a wide array of beverages and beverage mixes with added vitamin C, from Tang to cranberry juice cocktail. Milk has added vitamin D. Enrichment of food is common. But enrichment with pantothenic acid is not.

Losses of Pantothenic Acid

By the time ordinary, all-purpose white flour gets to your supermarket, whether in the form of the flour itself or as bread, cookies, or pasta, it has lost about half of the pantothenic acid it had as unprocessed wheat. Mill feed, the part of the wheat left over after the white flour is removed, has four and a half times as much pantothenic acid as the flour and is also very high in other vitamins that have been lost during milling, including B_1, B_2, niacin, B_6, folic acid, and vitamin E. Mill feed, as its name implies, is fed to animals (Schroeder 1971).

White rice has also lost half its pantothenic acid through milling. Cake flour has lost even more, as has precooked rice. Rye bread has lost two thirds of the pantothenic acid of the unprocessed grain (Schroeder 1971).

Studies of ready-to-eat breakfast cereals have shown that, in general, they contain very little pantothenic acid. Even the cereals made from whole wheat, which still has the bran and the germ attached to it (Shredded Wheat, Wheaties, Wheat Chex), and which could be expected to have high amounts of pantothenic acid, have lost 20 to 30 percent of the pantothenic acid from the original wheat. Corn flakes and puffed rice have lost about 65 percent of the pantothenic acid in raw corn and unmilled rice. Cheerios seem to have the highest amount of naturally-occurring pantothenic acid by a substantial margin, about twice as much, weight for weight, as Shredded Wheat (Schroeder 1971, Walsh, 1981).

But what do these figures mean in terms of the Daily Value? For some comparisons among breakfast cereals, look at Table 5.4.

Cereal	Serving Size	% Daily Value of Pantothenic Acid
Shredded Wheat	2 biscuits (46 g)	3.2%
Wheaties	1 cup (30 g)	2%
Corn Flakes	1 cup (30 g)	1%
Puffed Rice	1 cup (14 g)	0.5%
Cheerios	1 cup (30 g)	4%

(Sources: product labels; Schroeder 1971; Walsh 1981.)

Table 5.4 Comparison of Pantothenic Acid Content of Some Leading Cereals.

Now, returning to the natural wheat bread: 1 slice of whole wheat bread (36 g) provides about 2.7 percent of the Daily Value of pantothenic acid. (Those six slices the pyramid cites as good enough for the day contain some 16 percent.)

Clearly, unless breakfast cereals and bread are fortified with pantothenic acid, they are not important sources of the vitamin in an ordinary human diet. Bread is not fortified with it. And, as you might guess, none of the cereals in Table 5.4 are, either. (For a list of cereals that are, see Table 5.5.)

Cereal	% Daily Value
Kellogg's Product 19	100%
Kellogg's Healthy Choice	35%
Kellogg's Mueslix Crispy Blend	25%
Kellogg's Mueslix Apple & Almond Crunch	20%
GM Total	100%
GM Total Corn Flakes	100%
GM Total Raisin Bran	100%

Table 5.5 Seven Cereals Fortified With Pantothenic Acid.

But we eat more than just bread and cereal every day. What about the rest of our food?

Earlier, we said that some raw vegetables and broiled or baked meats were fairly good sources of pantothenic acid. But why raw, and why broiled or baked? The reason is that pantothenic acid is a water-soluble vitamin. This means that any processing that involves the food with water will leach out pantothenic acid. Cooking vegetables in water, steaming them, canning them, or freezing them (surely you've noticed all that ice in those packages!) all pull pantothenic acid out of the vegetables and into the water, which is usually discarded. If the cooking water is slightly acidic (if it contains lemon juice, vinegar, or tomatoes, for example) or alkaline (if it contains baking soda), the heat of cooking destroys the vitamin, and even drinking that water won't give it to you.

Losses of pantothenic acid in canning green vegetables average about 56 percent; in canning root vegetables, 46 percent; in canning peas and beans, 78 percent; in canning fruits and juices, 50 percent. Losses to freezing are around 50 percent in all vegetables, though only about 7 percent in fruits and juices (but these are already naturally low in pantothenic acid). Losses in cooking any of these foods, starting with the raw material, run as high as 44 percent. (Schroeder 1971).

Losses also occur in the processing of meat and seafood. Canning or freezing seafood results in about a 20 percent loss of pantothenic acid; canning meat about 26 percent. The amount lost when freezing meat has not been as well-established, but as an example, freezing beef tongue results in a 70 percent loss of pantothenic acid. Cooking meat or seafood by methods that involve adding water (stewing or braising) decreases their pantothenic acid content by one third to one half. Since broiling and baking free the least amount of water from the meat, they get rid of the least of the vitamin (Schroeder 1971).

So how much pantothenic acid do we really take in? Estimates of the typical American's consumption of this vitamin have varied from 5.8 to 11.5 mg per day. But according to an article in the *Journal of the American Dietetic Association* (Walsh 1981), these estimates of dietary intake have usually been based on raw food values. Given the significant losses of pantothenic acid in processing and cooking, the estimators have obviously been overjudging the amount of the vitamin that we consume, perhaps by as much as half. *The Handbook of Vitamins* (Fox 1984) suggests that, because of the increasing use of processed foods, people in industrial societies all over the world may not be getting enough pantothenic acid.

Can this be true, especially of Americans? When all our supermarket shelves are bulging with boxes, cans, bottles, and plastic-wrapped packages, could Americans possibly be malnourished? Sure we could.

WHAT WE EAT

We all know that we diet like crazy in America. We are obsessed with being thin, and we leap at the chance to try something that promises real weight loss. How else to explain the fanfare accompanying the introduction of that new non-digestible fat, Olestra? Non-fattening snack food—the dream of every dieter! But non-fat potato chips won't really save us from eating too much—or too much of the wrong things—at meals, so there is always another diet guru and another diet book waiting to help us to our goal. That goal is usually an alteration in our eating habits from unhealthy habits to healthy ones.

Let's choose a typical, best-selling diet book from the Health and Fitness section of our local bookstore. It looks like a sensible diet book, full of calorie and fat charts, suggested menus, tasty-looking low-fat recipes, and exercise advice. It seems likely that anyone following the author's suggestions, including a fourteen-day diet plan, would lose weight gradually without feeling starved.

As for the nutritional content of that diet plan—the author is a registered dietitian and presumably knows what she is talking about in this area. She notes that, over the fourteen days, the dieter's average daily intake of more than 25 vitamins and minerals would be at least 75 percent of the Recommended Daily Allowance, and in most cases more than the RDA. (Remember, the RDA for vitamins is the same as the Daily Value.) Even so, she endorses supplementing this diet with daily multivitamins, "for insurance."

Is the amount of pantothenic acid in this diet plan closer to 75 percent of the Daily Value, or closer to 100 percent? The author doesn't say (she doesn't list any specific vitamin

Food Source	Pantothenic Acid (mg)
Breakfast:	
1 ounce ready to eat cereal (Cheerios)	.38
1 cup bananas (5 oz)	.28
1 cup skim milk	.80
1 slice whole grain toast	.27
1 tsp light margarine	—
1 Tbs jelly or jam	.01
coffee or tea	—
Total breakfast pantothenic acid	1.74
Lunch:	
1 cup nonfat yogurt	.80
1 slice carrot-pineapple bread	.28
grapes (3.5 oz)	.20
no-cal beverage	—
Total lunch pantothenic acid	1.28
Dinner:	
3 oz flank steak	.72
1 baked potato (11 oz)	.99
1 cup broccoli (fresh, steamed, 3 oz)	.56
1 slice whole grain bread	.27
tossed vegetable salad (5 oz) (carrots, spinach, tomato)	.43
3 Tbs fat-free dressing	—
citrus fruit cup (4.5 oz)	.25
2 reduced-fat cookies	.12
no-cal beverage	—
Total dinner pantothenic acid	3.34
Total day's pantothenic acid	6.36

Table 5.6 A Published Daily Diet Plan

amounts for her diet plan), so let's take a look at one of her daily menus in terms of its pantothenic acid content (Table 5.6).

All amounts of the vitamin were calculated on the basis of charts from the *Journal of the American Dietetic Association* (Walsh 1981) and *The American Journal of Clinical Nutrition* (Schroeder 1971), and also the label from Carnation Non-Fat Dry Milk. The individual ingredients of her recipe for carrot-pineapple bread were used for calculating its pantothenic acid content. Where she did not specify weights, actual portions of food were weighed. Total calories, according to this book, 1,480.

This menu squares pretty well with the Food Pyramid; it's certainly low enough in milk and meat, and as compensation, it's high in fruits and vegetables. Lunch seems a little light, but the rest looks satisfying enough. Unfortunately, it only provides 63.6 percent of the RDA/Daily Value for pantothenic acid. You would certainly be well-advised to add that multivitamin with this diet.

Now let's look at a more ordinary day's food, no dieting this time around, but rather a substantial (and maybe even slightly excessive) 2,300 calories. An amount of food that would require a little exercise to work off. (Calories calculated from the diet book and from food labels. Weights and pantothenic acid content as before.) It starts with a good breakfast, which your mother always said was important, goes on to a fast-food lunch, and ends with a satisfying dinner, though without dessert (see Table 5.7).

As far as the Food Pyramid goes, this is, of course, much more from the meat/poultry/eggs section than is recommended, and not enough fruits and vegetables. And in spite of its large number of calories, it, too, falls short of the Daily Value of pantothenic acid, with only 76.4 percent. So how do these two diets compare to yours, or to the average American diet?

In 1977, researchers at the Clayton Foundation Biochemical Institute of the University of Texas at Austin evaluated the average American diet, using information on American food consumption from the U.S. Department of Agriculture.

Food Source	Pantothenic Acid (mg)
Breakfast:	
2 eggs (4 oz)	1.22
2 slices whole wheat toast	.55
2 Tbs jelly	.02
1 cup skim milk	.80
1 cup fruit (5 oz)	.28
Total breakfast pantothenic acid	2.87
Lunch:	
1 hamburger bun	.20
4 oz burger with 1 oz cheese	.84
lettuce	—
1 slice tomato (2.5 oz)	.23
1 Tbs mustard	—
1 oz potato chips	.20
no-cal beverage	—
Total lunch pantothenic acid	1.43
Dinner:	
1/2 tomato (3.5 oz)	.33
1 carrot (2 oz)	.16
1/2 cup broccoli (1.5 oz)	.50
lettuce	—
2 Tbs lowfat French dressing	—
1 French roll	.20
1 Tbs butter	—
6 oz chicken	2.02
1 cup Rice-a-Roni	.13
no-cal beverage	—
Total dinner pantothenic acid	3.34
Total day's pantothenic acid	7.64

Table 5.7 An Average American One-Day 2,300 Calorie Menu, Including Fast-Food Lunch.

As far as vitamins were concerned, they found this average diet to be much too low in biotin, vitamin E, folic acid, vitamin K, and pantothenic acid (Williams 1987).

The truth is that it's hard to eat a diet that meets the Daily Value for pantothenic acid unless you focus on the relatively small number of foods that are high in the vitamin (see Table 5.1 again). A serving of liver every day would certainly do the trick, if that appealed to you. But otherwise, modern food processing just doesn't leave enough pantothenic acid in our food to enable us to reach the Daily Value just through normal eating.

So, the accepted wisdom that anyone who eats a well-balanced diet doesn't need vitamin supplements turns out to be a myth. What to do, then? Multivitamin pills are one option; they usually provide 100 percent of the Daily Value. Liquid supplements like Ensure are another (25 percent of the Daily Value). And those seven cereals fortified with pantothenic acid (Table 5.5) are a third (20 percent to 100 percent of the Daily Value). Or, you can add a vitamin-rich powdered flavoring to your milk, like Ovaltine Rich Chocolate (25 percent of the Daily Value, if you include the skim milk; but note that the other flavors of Ovaltine do not contain pantothenic acid).

Now we're left with one last question about that Daily Value. Is it really enough?

IS THE DAILY VALUE ENOUGH?

The Daily Value/RDA for pantothenic acid is 10 mg. But if you read the FDA's own *Recommended Dietary Allowances, 10th Edition* (1989—the most recent), you'll realize that the figure is just a guess. It's an educated guess, based on how much pantothenic acid is in the self-selected diets of apparently healthy people, and on how much seems to cycle through the healthy human body each day, but still, just a guess. *Recommended Dietary Allowances* actually says that the

FDA subcommittee studying pantothenic acid decided that there was insufficient evidence for setting a daily requirement for adults (although it did recommend a provisional amount for children of 2 to 3 mg, based on the pantothenic acid content of human milk). In spite of that, charts of the RDAs in issues of *FDA Consumer* magazine, as long ago as 1979 and as recently as 1993, show pantothenic acid with an RDA or a Daily Value of 10 mg.

Should It Be Different?

In this context, it is interesting to note that our old friends, the laboratory rats, only did well when their daily intake of pantothenic acid was .02 mg or more. Less than that, and they showed symptoms of deficiency, they grew poorly, and they died prematurely. It is, of course, chancy to generalize from rats to human beings; there are many ways in which rats are not like us. But it is worth observing that .02 mg of pantothenic acid for a 45g rat is equivalent to 30 mg for a 150 pound human being—three times the Daily Value.

HUMAN VARIABILITY

We are not all the same. We know that, of course. We know that no two people have the same fingerprints. We know that some people are allergic to pollen or mold, some to certain foods, like chocolate or milk or strawberries, some to animals or their products, like wool, feathers, or fur. Some people break out in hives if they take sulfa or prednisone, and some go into shock or even die from bee stings or penicillin shots. And these are only a few of the ways in which we differ from each other, there are countless others. Each of us is a physical and chemical individual, with our own individual reactions to foods, medicines, and our surroundings.

This human variability is well-recognized in scientific research, and is one reason why scientists try to use a large number of subjects in any study. With a large number of subjects, both the commonly-occurring and the relatively rare effects can be observed and weighed against each other.

For example, when a new drug is tested, the researchers don't expect every test subject to react to it in the same way. When diclofenac (Voltaren), a frequently-prescribed non-steroidal anti-inflammatory drug, or NSAID, was initially tested on human beings, some of the test subjects experienced unpleasant side effects. 20 percent of them had gastrointestinal symptoms like diarrhea, indigestion, nausea, or constipation, 7 percent got headaches, and 3 percent experienced dizziness. Various other symptoms, such as fluid retention, rashes, and ringing in the ears occurred among 1–3 percent of subjects. Looking at these numbers from the opposite point of view, however, we can see this research showed that 80 percent of the subjects had no gastrointestinal problems, 93 percent had no headaches, 97 percent did not get dizzy, and 97–99 percent did not retain fluids or develop rashes or ringing in the ears. These numbers mean that diclofenac is worth trying when a strong NSAID is called for, because the majority of people don't experience these side effects. So, if you happen to be a person who, because of natural human variability, does experience unpleasant side effects, you can switch to some other NSAID in the hope that you'll have better luck with it. (See Chapter Three for more on NSAIDs.)

In the pantothenic acid deficiency studies discussed in Chapter Four, the researchers noted that the principle of great variation among normal people was amply demonstrated in their work. Though there were broad similarities in the volunteers' responses to a lack of the vitamin, every man also showed some individual symptoms that were not duplicated in any of the others. For example, only one of the volunteers experienced burning feet (previously recognized as the most obvious symptom of the deficiency), and only one developed an odd goose-stepping way of walking (previously observed only in pantothenic acid-deficient pigs).

Knowing about human variability, what can we say about the Daily Value for any vitamin, let alone pantothenic acid? Remember, the Daily Value is supposed to represent the highest amount of a vitamin that most people need each day. Is it possible that some people have a higher requirement for some vitamins?

Dr. Roger J. Williams, discoverer of pantothenic acid, researched and wrote about vitamins, nutrition, and medicine for more than forty years. He was also a pioneer in the study of human variability with his book, *Biochemical Individuality* (1956). He suggested that the human need for pantothenic acid could vary substantially from person to person. He himself took vitamin and mineral supplements that included 15 mg of pantothenic acid (one and a half times the Daily Value), and he believed that this would be a good "insurance" level for all Americans, given the poor nutritional values of the typical American diet. He also thought that some people might even require much larger doses—"megadoses"—of any or all of the B vitamins and vitamin C, depending on their own individual body chemistries.

Perhaps most importantly, Williams noted that it was clear from animal research that animals could have pantothenic acid deficiencies that ranged from mild to severe, and in the mild deficiencies the animals often looked fairly healthy. The possible existence of mild pantothenic acid deficiencies in human beings, he thought, had not been adequately investigated. (For more about his research, see Chapters Four and Six.)

In the case of pantothenic acid and what the human body does with it, the concept of individual variation is certainly borne out by scientific research. For example, a 1951 study of 96 people who were given identical injections of the vitamin showed that, over the following twenty-four hours, they flushed out widely varying amounts of it in their urine—some of them getting rid of up to twice as much as others. And in a 1981 study of 77 subjects, blood levels of pantothenic acid varied considerably from one person to another, even though their diets were similar.

Can we combine human variability with an inadequate level of pantothenic acid in the average diet and come to the conclusion that some people may be at least mildly deficient in the vitamin? Let's look at another element in this equation first.

THE STONE AGE DIET

Human beings did not evolve eating bread. For about the last ten thousand years, most human beings have been farmers, living primarily on grain products, and raising some fruits, vegetables, and meat animals on the side, sometimes with a little fish thrown in. In relatively recent times, in some places (like the United States), meat has become the center of our diet, but throughout a great deal of the world, bread (or pasta, or rice) is still the staff of life. The Food Pyramid, after all, calls for more servings of grain foods per day than of any other category. That is considered proper nutrition.

But ten thousand years is not a very long time in the life of the human species. For over a million and a half years before that, our Stone Age ancestors were hunters and gatherers, not farmers. They killed and ate wild animals, and they foraged for edible wild vegetation—fruits, vegetables, nuts, and roots. They rarely, if ever, ate grains. This diet, not the farmers' diet, is the one the human race is really adapted to.

After examining the diets of the few groups of hunters and gatherers left in the modern world (like the !Kung of the Kalahari and the Australian Aborigines), Eaton and Konner (1985) made some important observations on the nutritional levels of pre-agricultural human beings. Compared to our modern American diet, that Stone Age diet was much healthier—lower in fat and sodium, higher in protein, fiber, and calcium, and substantially higher in all vitamins. As a vitamin sample, Konner and Eaton calculated the amount of vitamin C in the Stone Age diet; it came out to 392 mg, or six and a half times the present Daily Value of 60 mg. Konner and Eaton also noted that because the Stone Age diet was high in meat (20 to 35 percent of the total daily food intake), it was also high in iron, vitamin B_{12}, and folic acid.

With such a high-meat diet (about one and three quarter pounds per day), and also because our Stone Age ancestors undoubtedly ate the tenderest parts of the animals, the organ meats (highest in pantothenic acid), their pantothenic acid intake would also have been significantly higher than our current Daily Value.

The change in our diet—from a high-meat diet that also included a wide variety of vegetable foods to a limited, high-grain (and milled grain, at that) diet—resulted in various deficiency diseases that we have only begun to come to terms with in the last 250 years. Scurvy (lack of vitamin C), the first deficiency disease to be recognized as such, was first treated in 1753; beriberi (lack of B_1) was recognized as a deficiency disease in the late Nineteenth Century, pellagra (lack of niacin) in 1937. We have only recently begun to recognize folic acid deficiency. Should pantothenic acid deficiency be added to the list? Before we can make a final decision on that, we need to take a closer look at pantothenic acid in our bodies and at the Daily Value itself.

PANTOTHENIC ACID STORED IN OUR BODIES

In Chapter Four, we saw how important pantothenic acid is to our lives. We saw that in its stripped down form (the pure vitamin) it circulates in the blood, and in its more complex form (coenzyme A) it occurs in every organ of the body. This is, of course, because every part of the body has a use for it. How much pantothenic acid are we talking about here?

Table 5.8 shows the amounts of pantothenic acid found in some of the tissues of a typical healthy mammal body. It also shows average weights (and in the case of blood, an average volume) of these tissues in human beings, based on a total body weight of 150 pounds. For the sake of simplicity, the figure for skeletal muscle represents an average of male and female values (in general, men have more muscle in proportion to their total body weights than women).

Amounts of pantothenic acid in various mammal tissues, and average weights of those tissues (or volume, in the case of blood) in a 150-pound human being. A 150-pound human being weighs 68,000 g.

TISSUE	PANTOTHENIC ACID IN TISSUE	WEIGHT OF TISSUE	PANTOTHENIC ACID TOTAL
Liver	75 mcg/g	1,350 g	101,250 mcg or 101.2 mg
Heart	20 mcg/g	255 g	5,100 mcg or 5.1 mg
Brain	18 mcg/g	1,335 g	24,030 mcg or 24.0 mg
Kidney	45 mcg/g	280 g	12,600 mcg or 12.6 mg
Skeletal muscle	9.9 mcg/g	26,325 g	260,618 mcg or 260.6 mg
Blood	1.077 mcg/ml	4,500 ml*	4846 mcg or 4.8 mg
TOTAL PANTOTHENIC ACID IN ABOVE TISSUES:			408.3 mg

A microgram ("mcg") is one millionth of a gram, and a milliliter ("ml") is one thousandth of a liter (a liter is a little more than a quart). "Mcg/g" means micrograms of pantothenic acid per gram of tissue.

*Blood is measured in volume.

(Sources: Novelli 1953; Barton-Wright and Elliott 1963; Nourse 1964; Sherlock 1974.)

Table 5.8 Pantothenic Acid in Mammal Tissue.

Using these figures, we can estimate the minimum amount of pantothenic acid that must be present at any one time in the body of a healthy 150-pound person. It's a minimum estimate because we don't know pantothenic acid levels for other important tissues, like the lungs and intestines, that certainly contain the vitamin (all tissues do), but it will give us a ball-park figure. As you can see from Table 5.8, that figure is about 400 mg.

If we add in the approximately 9.5 percent of body weight that represents the rest of the internal organs (about 14 pounds for a 150-pound person) and assume that it has the same vitamin level as skeletal muscle (probably an underestimate, judging from the other internal organs), we have an additional 64 mg of pantothenic acid. This would raise our estimate to around 470 mg.

This is the approximate amount that is stored in the human body. At an excretion rate of between 1 and 7 mg per day (with an average of 3.75 mg) no wonder the deficiency studies took so long to show results! And no wonder the volunteers, deprived of the vitamin and then given large supplements in Chapter Four didn't excrete very much of it—they were refilling that 470 mg reservoir.

Compared to the amount of pantothenic acid in our bodies, we take in a very small amount each day, and we flush an almost equal amount out. At those rates, it would take a very long time to seriously deplete our reserves. But it would also take a long time to build them back up again. As we have seen from this chapter, if anyone in the U.S. is suffering from a mild pantothenic acid deficiency, that person would not have an easy time reversing it simply by eating a "well-balanced diet." Such a deficiency would probably be a long-term situation, and its outward symptoms might appear minor, and might easily be attributed to other causes. Certainly, two of the major outward symptoms of the initial stages of human pantothenic acid deficiency are familiar enough to most of us—tiredness and irritability. In this modern, rush-rush world, neither of these is unusual.

WHO IS AT RISK OF DEFICIENCY?

In order to answer this question, we must first discuss the types of deficiency. There are two kinds of vitamin deficiencies: primary and secondary. A primary deficiency is caused when less of the vitamin is taken in than the body needs. If the Daily Value is our measure, many of us seem to be at least mildly deficient in pantothenic acid.

A secondary deficiency occurs when intake is adequate but, due to some other factor, the body isn't able to use it all. For example, the vitamin may not be absorbed properly. People with chronic ulcerative or granulomatous colitis are likely to become deficient because their diseased intestinal tissues block the conversion of pantothenic acid into its active form, coenzyme A. Alcoholics may become deficient because alcohol decreases the amount of the vitamin in the tissues, where it is stored and does its job.

People who have abnormally low or high excretion levels of the vitamins are at risk, too. A too-low excretion level may mean that the body is hoarding its supplies because too little is coming in. A too-high excretion level (in cases where the person is not taking vitamin supplements) may mean that too much of the vitamin is being flushed out of the body, and reserves may be in danger of being lowered. A study of oral contraceptive users showed that they have lower than normal excretion levels of pantothenic acid. Studies of diabetics (diabetes mellitus) show that they have higher than normal excretion levels.

According to the *Handbook of Vitamins* (Fox 1984), all of the above groups are at risk for pantothenic acid deficiency.

A 1960 study of people with rheumatoid arthritis showed that this group excreted abnormally high levels of pantothenic acid. It seems obvious that they, too, must be at risk for the deficiency. We'll get back to this very significant fact in the next chapter, when we take a look at the research into arthritis and pantothenic acid. But first let's take another look at the Daily Value and what it means.

THE CHANGING RDA

Our understanding of vitamins has grown gradually over the last sixty years, and in that time scientists have changed their minds several times about the amount of vitamins that we really need in our daily diet. Table 5.9 compares the Recommended Daily Allowances of various vitamins in 1945, 1967, and 1993.

You'll notice on Table 5.9 that some vitamins are measured in I.U. (International Units) rather than in milligrams or micrograms. The I.U. is a measure of vitamin activity, not of weight. It is generally used for the oil-soluble vitamins A, D, E, and K because each of them occurs in several different forms, and these forms do not all have the same vitamin activity per unit of weight. Thus, 1 I.U. of retinol (vitamin A) weighs .3 mcg, while 1 I.U. of beta-carotene (which our bodies transform into vitamin A) weighs .6 mcg, but both behave in our bodies as exactly the same amount of vitamin A.

Even today, there is controversy over what the proper levels of some vitamins should be. Many medical scientists are recommending very high doses of the vitamins E, C, and beta-carotene. These vitamins seem to help protect against a host of diseases, including cancer, heart disease, and cataracts. They may even delay some of the effects of aging.

The *University of California at Berkeley Wellness Letter* suggests 200 to 800 I.U. of vitamin E a day, 250 to 500 mg of vitamin C, and 6 to 15 mg of beta-carotene (equal to 10,000 to 25,000 I.U. of vitamin A). As you can see, these figures are far higher than the RDAs/Daily Values of these vitamins. (Beta-carotene is recommended instead of vitamin A itself because vitamin A is toxic in high doses. See Chapter Eight for more on high doses of vitamin A and beta-carotene.)

The whole field of vitamin research is in a state of flux these days. A few years from now, the list of Daily Values may look quite different from that 1993 roster.

The following table compares RDAs for an average man in 1945, 1967, and 1993.

Vitamin	1945	1945	1967	1993
	SEDENTARY LIFESTYLE 2500 cal.	MODERATELY ACTIVE 3000 cal.		
B1	1.2 mg	1.5 mg	1.2 mg	1.5 mg
B2	1.6 mg	2.0 mg	1.7 mg	1.7 mg
B6	unknown	unknown	1.5 mg	2 mg
B12	X	X	3-5 mcg	6 mcg
Niacin	12 mg	15 mg	19 mg	20 mg
Biotin	unknown	unknown	.002–.003 mg	.3 mg
Folic acid	unknown	unknown	.15 mg	.4 mg
Panto. acid	unknown	unknown	10 mg	10 mg
C	75 mg	75 mg	70 mg	60 mg
D	sunlight	sunlight	unknown	400 I.U.
E	unknown	unknown	10–30 I.U.	30 I.U.

(Sources: *Encyclopaedia Britannica Book of the Year*, 1946; Sebrell and Haggerty 1967; *FDA Consumer Magazine*, Nov. 1993.) X means the vitamin had not yet been discovered. The 1945 figures are for a 154 lb. man and specify lifestyle and calorie intake per day. The 1967 and 1993 figures do not specify weight, gender, lifestyle, or calorie intake.

Table 5.9 The RDAs of Various Vitamins.

OTHER VITAMIN USES

If we choose—and many of us do, perhaps even without thinking about it—vitamins can play additional roles in our lives.

There are other medical uses for them, either already established or under research. Megadoses of niacin are sometimes prescribed to lower cholesterol, although the possible side effects (the intense flushing of the so-called "niacin rush," irregular heartbeat, or liver damage) can make that impractical. Some scientists think that vitamin D may reduce the risk of osteoporosis, and that folic acid (a very active area of research these days) may reduce the risk of colon and cervical cancer.

There are also cosmetic uses of vitamins. Who hasn't heard of the vitamin A anti-wrinkle creams? Formerly, such creams were prescribed to treat acne, but in recent times they achieved a new popularity because they can eliminate superficial wrinkles. In fact, if you look on the labels of many face creams, you will find various vitamins listed, including A, C, and E, although in past times no claims were made for any of them. And then there is para-aminobenzoic acid (PABA), not exactly a vitamin, but often lumped in with the B vitamins in nutritional supplements. When its capacity as a sunscreen was noticed, it suddenly became an ingredient in a very large number of facial cosmetics.

From our point of view, though, the most interesting use of vitamins outside the arena of nutrition is in shampoo and hair conditioners. Pantene was the first brand name to advertise its use of "provitamin B_5," and it apparently drew its name from the vitamin. Because vitamins are not patentable, any company could include them in their ingredients, and so you can now find this substance in a wide variety of hair care products. It is generally listed on the label as "panthenol." As you may have guessed, it is a form of pantothenic acid, in this case the alcohol version, which is equivalent to the vitamin.

You may already be using pantothenic acid supplements—on your hair! Unfortunately, no matter how good the vitamin may be for your hair, it doesn't get inside your body this way.

PANTOTHENIC ACID CONCLUSIONS

In this chapter, we have seen that the so-called well-balanced diet does not provide the Recommended Daily Allowance/ Daily Value of pantothenic acid because of losses of the vitamin in processing and cooking. We have also seen that the Daily Value itself is not hard and fast and that it may indeed be too low, at least for some people. And we have noted that people with one form of arthritis—rheumatoid—may be among those at risk for mild deficiency.

Now let's go on and see, in the next chapter, what the scientific research on arthritis and pantothenic acid can tell us.

Chapter 6

THE PREVIOUS RESEARCH

Before 1994, only a small amount of research had been done on the connection between pantothenic acid and arthritis, and none of it in the United States. In this chapter, we'll take a look at this research and see what it has to tell us. But first we'll examine some other scientific evidence that may point in the same direction, and we'll ask a few questions about what this evidence means. Finally, we'll look at other research on pantothenic acid that has additional implications for our lives and our health.

PANTOTHENIC ACID AND HEALING

By the early 1980s, there were a number of reports of pantothenic acid's healing properties. Good results had been obtained in healing bed sores and varicose ulcers (open sores, especially around the ankles, caused by varicose veins) by applying the vitamin externally, directly to the affected areas (Marks 1975). Minor skin irritation and itching had also been treated successfully with topical application of the vitamin. (Otrokov 1977, Moiseenok 1981)

In 1982, a group of doctors in Strasbourg, France, began investigating the use of pantothenic acid supplements in healing wounds (Grenier 1982, Aprahamian 1985). Using rabbits for their research, they determined that giving the animals injections of the vitamin made wounds heal faster than normal in the skin, in the large intestine, and in a tendon-like connective tissue called aponeurosis. In 1995, they recruited a group of human volunteers who were having tattoos removed and observed that a combination of pantothenic acid (although only one-seventh the amount they had given the rabbits) and vitamin C also had a positive effect on healing (Vaxman 1995).

Skin (site of the bed sores, the varicose ulcers, the irritation, the itching, some of the rabbit wounds, and the tattoos) and aponeurosis are both connective tissues—the materials that support our bodies and give it form. As we noted in Chapter Two, many kinds of arthritis are diseases of connective tissue.

Several researchers have pointed out that because pantothenic acid is essential to the formation of two important components of connective tissue, a deficiency of the vitamin would lead to a shortage of those substances. This in turn might cause what the researchers refer to as "abnormalities" in that tissue (Novelli 1953, Welsh 1954). Could such abnormalities contribute to arthritis? Could damage to the connective tissue that cannot be repaired because of the shortage of those two substances lead to arthritis?

PANTOTHENIC ACID AND FATIGUE

Fatigue is an important factor in many kinds of arthritis, and as we saw in Chapter Four, it is the earliest and most obvious symptom of pantothenic acid deficiency. Research done in the 1960s indicated that supplements of thiamine plus pantothenic acid decreased the fatigue and increased the endurance of exercising athletes. A 1985 study showed that pantothenic acid alone was also effective in this capacity (Williams 1989, Heiby 1988).

As we also saw in Chapter Four, pantothenic acid is at the heart of the body's major energy production. Do these studies mean that pantothenic acid can provide extra energy when the body needs it? And is there perhaps some implication here, not just for arthritis but also for chronic fatigue syndrome?

PANTOTHENIC ACID AND PHYSICAL STRESS

Again in Chapter Four, we saw that pantothenic acid enables the body's adrenal glands to manufacture steroid hormones. One of these hormones—cortisone—is essential in times of physical stress such as infection, surgery, lowered oxygen levels (as at high altitudes), or exposure to cold. Without it, such stresses can cause a person to collapse and even die. People with Addison's disease have adrenal glands that don't make enough steroid hormones, and they must be supplemented with synthetic hormones, especially with cortisone; and in times of stress, their cortisone dosages are raised to prevent collapse.

Supplements of pantothenic acid have been shown to increase a human being's ability to withstand the stress of being immersed in cold water (Heiby 1988). And of course, the exercise discussed in the preceding section was also a stress, and supplements of the vitamin allowed the subjects to withstand it better. If stress requires cortisone, do these studies mean that extra pantothenic acid enables the body to make extra amounts of its own natural cortisone when necessary?

We know that cortisone can help arthritis. Is it possible that pantothenic acid can fight arthritis with the body's own natural cortisone?

PUTTING THESE CLUES TOGETHER

Healing connective tissue, decreasing fatigue, making cortisone—pantothenic acid has been shown to do all these things. And they all have some association with arthritis. At this point we may have some suspicions, but we can't let ourselves jump to any conclusions on the basis of this kind of indirect evidence. We have to look at the research done directly on pantothenic acid and arthritis.

Pantothenic Acid and Rheumatoid Arthritis

In Finland in 1960, a team of researchers was studying the excretion of four B vitamins (B_1, B_2, niacin, and pantothenic acid) in the urine of thirty people who had rheumatoid arthritis (Kalliomaki 1960). They discovered that, although excretion of the first three vitamins was below normal levels in a few of their subjects, excretion of pantothenic acid was above normal in all of them. People with rheumatoid arthritis were dumping pantothenic acid out of their bodies very fast.

What does this mean? In Chapter Five we noted that people who excreted high amounts of pantothenic acid, but were not taking supplements, were at risk of deficiency. Could this be true of people with rheumatoid arthritis?

With high excretion levels, one might also expect low blood levels, since pantothenic acid leaves the blood to be excreted in the urine. In England in 1963, two researchers (Barton-Wright and Elliott 1963) reported that levels of pantothenic acid in the blood of sixty-six people with rheumatoid arthritis were much lower than normal. And the lower their pantothenic acid levels were, the worse their arthritis symptoms were. To investigate what seemed to be an obvious relationship, the researchers decided to try supplementing twenty of their subjects with daily injections of pantothenic acid.

After seven days, pantothenic acid levels in the subjects' blood had risen to normal and their arthritis symptoms had been alleviated. And through the next three weeks, as the daily injections were continued, they stayed that way. Then the injections were stopped and gradually, over the course of a month, their pantothenic acid levels sank back to where they had started from, and their arthritis symptoms returned.

Pantothenic Acid and Osteoarthritis

After seeing the report by Barton-Wright and Elliot, which was published in the prestigious British medical journal *The Lancet*, another British researcher (Annand 1963) wrote to the magazine to tell about his own research, which had been published in a different journal the previous year (Annand 1962).

It seemed that, in his reading, Dr. Annand had come across an article from 1950 about bone development in rats that were pantothenic acid deficient, and he had been struck by how similar the rats' bone deformities were to osteoarthritis. As a result, he began treating his osteoarthritis patients with supplements of the vitamin. Within fourteen days of starting the supplements (which in this case were pills, not shots), twenty of twenty-six patients showed significant improvement. Subsequently, ten of these successes discontinued their pantothenic acid and their symptoms returned, only to improve again after they restarted the vitamin.

In 1967, Barton-Wright and Elliot took up the challenge of osteoarthritis and successfully treated more than 40 osteoarthritis patients with a combination of pantothenic acid and cysteine, a substance that the body can convert into a component of connective tissue. (By this time, they, too, had switched to pills.) Then two more British researchers (Haslock and Wright 1971) tested the combination of pantothenic acid and cysteine on forty people with osteoarthritis in their knees and found that didn't work any better than a placebo did. (A placebo is a pill that doesn't have the active ingredient being tested.)

Follow-up to the British Studies

In 1971, the situation was looking pretty confused. Pantothenic acid, either alone or in combination with cysteine, had worked for some subjects and for some researchers, but not for others. And although three sets of researchers had worked on osteoarthritis (two of them successfully), only one had dealt with rheumatoid arthritis; there had been no follow-up on that.

Science requires that research be followed up, repeated, and confirmed. A single positive study cannot be conclusive. It can only point the way, raise questions, and suggest further research. In Chapter Ten, we'll talk about why there has been so little follow-up on the arthritis-pantothenic acid connection. For now, though, we'll look at the last British study that came out of all of this previous research, a study done in 1980.

That year, twenty-two members of the General Practitioner Research Group—doctors scattered all over Great Britain—published their own study of pantothenic acid and arthritis. Coordinating their efforts, they had recruited ninety-four subjects with various forms of arthritis, but mainly osteoarthritis and rheumatoid arthritis. They had administered the vitamin only (without cysteine), in pill form, and in much higher dosages than any of the earlier studies. For osteoarthritis, their results were negative—the vitamin didn't help. But in patients with rheumatoid arthritis, the vitamin caused a significant reduction in pain and stiffness. The doctors ended their article by calling for more research to confirm that latter effect (General Practitioner Research Group 1980).

That was where research on pantothenic acid and arthritis stood in the English-speaking world in 1980. In 1984, an article reviewing vitamin therapy in general cited most of the articles we've talked about and also called for more research on the pantothenic acid-arthritis connection (Ovesen 1984). But as of 1995, a search of the medical literature both in print and in computer databases showed that, in the world of English-language publishing, there seemed to be only one other article on the subject, and that was a translation of a study that originally appeared in a Russian-language journal published in the Soviet Union.

Let's take a look at it and at other related work that has been done in Eastern Europe.

THE ANTI-INFLAMMATORY PROPERTIES OF PANTOTHENIC ACID

Behind what used to be called the Iron Curtain, scientists have been studying the properties of pantothenic acid for more than thirty years. In the mid-1960s, researchers working at a children's hospital in Hungary became interested in its anti-inflammatory effects. They injected histamine under the skin of healthy children in order to provoke an allergic, inflammatory skin reaction (hives) and found that both oral and injected pantothenic acid reduced that inflammation (Szorady 1966).

In the Soviet Union in the 1970s, pantothenic acid was shown to reduce the inflammation of various skin diseases, including eczema, neurodermatitis (skin irritation caused by too much scratching), and allergic dermatoses (hives again) (Otrokov 1977, Moiseenok 1981). Indeed, according to Dr. Andrej Moiseenok of the Academy of Sciences of Belarus, who has been involved in pantothenic acid research for the past three decades, it is now widely used for such ailments in the former Soviet Union (Moiseenok 1994). But our interest is in internal inflammation, not in skin diseases.

The translated article was written by Dr. Moiseenok and ten colleagues, and it presented their research on pantothenic acid and adjuvant arthritis (Moiseenok 1981). Adjuvant arthritis is a form of arthritis caused by injecting an animal's joints with a substance (like formaldehyde) that provokes an immune response—that is, inflammation. After giving this form of arthritis to 140 rats, Dr. Moiseenok and his colleagues found that high doses of pantothenic acid reduced the inflammation substantially. The same experiment had been done by another group of scientists with the same results a few years earlier, but never published in English (Otrokov 1977).

For reasons we will discuss in Chapter Ten, this information from the former Soviet Union, and the countries once controlled by it, does not carry the kind of weight that American or Western European scientific research would. But there are American studies that support an anti-inflammatory effect for pantothenic acid—studies on lupus erythematosus.

In the early 1950s, researchers in the U.S. noted that people with lupus erythematosus excreted unusually high levels of pantothenic acid in their urine. Following familiar reasoning—that lupus is a connective tissue disease and pantothenic acid helps maintain connective tissue; that lupus can be treated with steroids, and pantothenic acid helps the adrenal glands make steroids—the researchers tried pantothenic acid on subjects with various forms of lupus. They focused on the various skin inflammations that are characteristic of the disease, hoping to reduce them, and their results were favorable enough to warrant further research.

In the follow-up, vitamin E was added to the pantothenic acid, because it, too, had shown some positive results in lupus, and also because vitamin E was known to boost the activities of other vitamins. The subjects took massive doses of both, far more pantothenic acid than in any other study we've looked at, though only about two to four times the vitamin E that some people now take routinely every day. (We'll talk more about dosages in Chapter Eight.) They also had to take these supplements for much longer before there were any observable results—from one to six months, depending on how bad their skin inflammations were and how long they had had them. But of the sixty-seven people treated with the combination of pantothenic acid and vitamin E, all improved, and in nearly half of them, the skin inflammations cleared up completely (Welsh 1954).

Because the focus of these studies was on skin inflammation, the question of arthritis—which, as we saw in Chapter Two, is one of the most common symptoms of lupus—was addressed only as a side issue. During the months of the major study, ten of the sixty-seven subjects did experience joint pain, and all responded well to sodium salicylate, an aspirin relative. That left fifty-seven subjects who did not experience joint pain.

To sum up what we've discovered so far: there is some evidence that pantothenic acid can reduce inflammation, both in the skin and in the joints. As we saw in Chapter Two, all forms of arthritis involve inflammation, but in rheumatoid arthritis the inflammation is especially great. Is this why Barton-Wright and Elliot and the General Practitioner Group got such consistent results in their rheumatoid arthritis subjects, while the results for osteoarthritis subjects were mixed at best? And is the vitamin's effect on joint inflammation why so few of the lupus subjects experienced one of their disease's most common symptoms during their months of treatment?

WHY DOES PANTOTHENIC ACID SEEM TO WORK FOR SOME ARTHRITIS?

The truth is that we don't know. Perhaps a mild, long-term pantothenic acid deficiency can cause arthritis. We know from Chapter Five that getting enough of the vitamin without taking supplements isn't easy. Perhaps some people have a higher requirement for the vitamin than others, either because they absorb less or because they dump it out of their bodies too fast, or because their metabolism simply uses more. Getting enough pantothenic acid just from food would be even harder for those people.

Perhaps some forms of arthritis can be caused by having too little pantothenic acid to properly maintain our connective tissue. Or perhaps some forms of arthritis have something to do with a shortage of our own natural cortisone, a potent anti-inflammatory. Does extra pantothenic acid promote extra manufacture of the body's own cortisone to combat inflammation? Or is pantothenic acid itself an anti-inflammatory, just another drug comparable to aspirin or ibuprofen?

We don't know. As Ovesen said in 1984, more research is called for. That's one reason why Dr. Scheiner and I did our own study of pantothenic acid and arthritis, which we'll talk about in Chapter Seven. But before we leave the topic of the previous research, there's a fascinating sidelight to explore.

PANTOTHENIC ACID AND LONGEVITY

As we said in Chapter Four, pantothenic acid, in its guise as coenzyme A, is a master enzyme of the body. It is involved in countless essential functions, from salt balance to energy production. It was inevitable, then, that Roger J. Williams, discoverer of pantothenic acid and advocate of nutritional supplements for everyone living in our modern, over-processed world, would look into what happened when otherwise healthy experimental animals were given supplements of his vitamin.

He knew two things before he started. First, that queen bees live far longer than worker bees—as long as seven years compared to the workers' mere weeks or months. And the food of the larva that is to become a queen is royal jelly, one of the richest natural sources of pantothenic acid that exists. Second, that fruit flies given drinking water laced with pantothenic acid lived 28 percent longer than fruit flies who drank plain water (Gardner 1948).

He chose mice as his experimental animals, because their lifespans are short, and the whole experiment could be finished in about two years. He divided the mice into two groups and fed them exactly the same controlled diet, except that one group had extra pantothenic acid in its water. The mice in the supplemented group lived 19 percent longer than the ones in the unsupplemented group (Williams 1958). As Williams pointed out, that's equivalent to thirteen human years.

As we mentioned earlier, Williams took extra pantothenic acid himself. In fact, he took a wide array of supplements, some of them at significantly higher levels than contained in the standard one-a-day type multivitamin. Dr. Williams lived to the age of 94 and was still active until two years before his death in 1988. (For his specific supplement formula, see his book *The Wonderful World Within You.*)

In this chapter we've learned that pantothenic acid can have a healing effect on wounds and inflammation, and that it can also help combat physical stress and fatigue. We've noted that people with rheumatoid arthritis have abnormal levels of pantothenic acid in their blood and urine, indicating that they may well be deficient in this vitamin. We've looked at the studies in England and Belarus that show pantothenic acid alleviating pain and inflammation in human beings and animals with various kinds of arthritis. And we've seen some evidence that pantothenic acid may even have life-extending potential.

Now let's move away from formal research for a while, from people who are just subjects and statistics, and find out what pantothenic acid has meant to the lives of some individual human beings who have joint pain.

Chapter 7

Our Research, Informal and Formal

There is anecdotal evidence for pantothenic acid's effect on arthritis. I've gathered a good deal of it myself. But that isn't proof. The human mind is powerful, and if a person expects something to help him, sometimes it will, even if there's no scientific or medical reason why it should. That is called the placebo effect.

On the other hand, as we've said before, we are all different, and what truly works for one person may not work for another. Scientific research is intended to distinguish between real effects, even if they don't happen to everyone, and placebo effects.

In this chapter, we will take a look at some of that anecdotal evidence, at the real stories of real people. And then we'll look at the formal, scientific study Dr. Scheiner and I did on pantothenic acid and arthritis.

SPREADING THE WORD ABOUT PANTOTHENIC ACID

For a long time after I started using pantothenic acid, I did not talk much about my arthritis. After all, it was just a tale of pain and misery past; I was doing fine, and no one would guess by watching me that there was anything wrong. I just took my vitamins every morning and didn't think about the joint pain that wasn't there any more. I didn't want to bore anybody with the details of what I had been through. And I didn't know anyone else who had arthritis—at least I thought I didn't—so the subject almost never came up in conversation.

Of course, I was wrong about not knowing anyone with arthritis. For years, I had no idea how common arthritis was. I didn't realize that plenty of other people had joint pain and were just as reticent as I was to talk about it. They coped one way or another, with pain pills or anti-inflammatories, or with exercise, or sometimes just by gritting their teeth and bearing it. But they didn't talk. My circle of friends was only that—friends, not an arthritis support group. On rare occasions I would tell someone about my experience with pantothenic acid, or my husband would, but no one ever came back to us to say they had tried it. I suspect that, like my own orthopedic surgeon, they thought it was just another quack cure.

About six years ago, though, all of that began to change. At a crowded Christmas party, where my husband and I had been circulating separately, he came up behind me, tapped me on the shoulder, and said, "You have to talk to Rosemary about pantothenic acid." That was the beginning of my quiet crusade on behalf of pantothenic acid, and the real first step on the road that led to this book.

Rosemary's Knee

Rosemary had arthroscopic surgery for a torn ligament in her right knee a little more than a year before the Christmas party. By the party—indeed, well before the party—she was supposed to have recovered, supposed to be able to walk without pain. But that hadn't happened, and her doctor couldn't give her any reason why. So there she was, leaning heavily on a cane when she had to move from one place to another, but mostly sitting in a single chair the whole evening, her face pale and drawn.

When I talked to her, she was in pain, and she was willing to try pretty much anything that held out the possibility of help. She was already taking Naprosyn, a strong NSAID, and it wasn't doing much good. She said she would start on pantothenic acid as soon as possible.

Although we had known Rosemary and her husband for nearly twenty years, we didn't see them very often; they lived out in the far suburbs, while we lived in the city. So it wasn't until a few months later, when they invited us to a party at their home, that I was able to observe the results of my advice.

Rosemary looked great. The cane was gone, and so was the pain in her knee. She was a smiling, attentive hostess, walking around the food-laden table as easily as any of her guests. She had been up since 5 o'clock that morning, getting everything ready for the party, and aside from pantothenic acid (which she still took regularly), she had needed only a single Anacin tablet. At 6 PM she was still going strong.

Within just a few days of starting the vitamin, she told me, she had been feeling much better. Six years later, she still takes pantothenic acid, though at a much lower dose—a maintenance dose—and she has almost no trouble with the knee.

Was it arthritis? Rosemary doesn't know; her doctor never called it that. But it was joint pain, and pantothenic acid got rid of virtually all of it.

Betty's Hands

It was at Betty's Christmas party that I found out about Rosemary's knee pain. Later, after Rosemary had such success with pantothenic acid, Betty decided to try it for her hands.

She was in her fifties, and for some time she had been having quite a lot of pain in her hands, especially in cold weather, or when there was a change in the weather or the temperature. Even gripping the cold steering wheel of her car would bring on extreme pain. The joints of her fingers were also beginning to bend sideways. She had been diagnosed with osteoarthritis.

She started with a lower dose of the vitamin than Rosemary had, and she added vitamin E on her own. It took three or four months for her to notice any effect, but finally the pain went away, and her fingers even straightened out. She believes the vitamin E worked with the pantothenic acid to cause her improvement.

At one point, after she had been feeling much better for a while, Betty decided she was tired of taking so many pills, and she discontinued her vitamin supplements. After two or three weeks without them, the pain in her hands came back, and she went back to her vitamins.

Like Rosemary, she now takes a lower, maintenance dose of pantothenic acid. If her hands bother her a little occasionally (and it doesn't happen very often), she takes aspirin. She says that if the old pain came back, she wouldn't hesitate to up her dosage of pantothenic acid.

Pat's Knees

I met Pat on the Internet when I was trying to recruit volunteers for the study that Dr. Scheiner and I wanted to run. For various reasons, she couldn't volunteer, but she was willing to try pantothenic acid on her own.

Pat was diagnosed with rheumatoid arthritis about ten years ago, when she was twenty-seven. She also had osteoarthritis in her knees as a result of old injuries. She had achy hands and quite a lot of knee pain, which got worse with changes in the weather. She was especially bothered by it when going up and down stairs—the pains were like knives stabbing under her kneecaps.

She started taking pantothenic acid in late April or early May of 1994. By the end of June, she was noticing a definite decrease in her discomfort—her aches and pains in general were less, even when the weather changed. By late August, she was doing better than she had in years; she could go up and down stairs without any pain. In May of 1995, she sent me excited electronic mail—she had gone dancing, something she hadn't done in quite a long time, and there was no pain in her knees at all.

Pat continues to take pantothenic acid, and her pains are rare these days. At last report she was able to run two blocks to catch a bus, and without any pain.

Dave's Knee

Dave's pain and stiffness, which were primarily in his left knee and to a smaller degree in his left ankle, were from an old injury—he had been struck by a car in 1993. Because his job required a lot of walking, he felt the pain much of the time, and he thought of it as being very much like a toothache pain.

He started taking pantothenic acid in March of 1995, and noticed an effect after two or three weeks. By the end of April, although the stiffness in his knee was still there, the pain had diminished to almost nothing. Now, after too much walking or other exertion (like pushing a car to help someone), the knee gets stiff and sometimes even swells up, but the toothache pain is gone. He doesn't complain at all about the ankle.

Dave continues to take pantothenic acid.

Mark's Back

Sixteen years ago, when he was 25, Mark fell off the roof while servicing his ham radio antenna. He hurt his back at the time, but it wasn't very bad, and he seemed to recover fully. Two years later, though, he started to experience intense pain in his back, pain that would come back every autumn and last for weeks at a time before finally fading away. Eventually, it got so bad that, during a flare, he could not even dress himself.

His doctor X-rayed his back and said the trouble must have been caused by some kind of injury. It was at that point that Mark made the connection with his tumble off the roof. The doctor called his condition "degenerative arthritis" (we know it as osteoarthritis) and told him to rest and take prescription NSAIDs. That helped a little over the years, but not really enough, and the NSAIDs always made him tired.

The pain came back every two or three years, and Mark took NSAIDs for it, although he wasn't satisfied with them. They helped, he said, but they weren't great. In 1995, when the pain struck, he took them for two weeks. Then, because he had heard about pantothenic acid from mutual friends, he stopped the NSAIDs and switched to the vitamin. Between pantothenic acid and a heating pad, the pain went away after a week.

Larry's Back

Larry's low back pain started when he was twenty or twenty-one years old and in the navy. Later, when he was in his thirties and working in theater, he lifted a heavy piece of scenery and herniated a disk. He also has scoliosis (a gradual twisting of the spine). The result of all of this is that although his back is fine for months at a time, sometimes, especially when he overstrains it by hunching over a computer for ten or twelve hours at a stretch, the pain is severe. Formerly, when the pain was very bad, he took Doan's pills or Tylenol, but neither of them helped him a lot.

Larry decided to try pantothenic acid for one of his flares, and within a short time he felt better and no longer needed to take painkillers as often as before. But because he was feeling better, he stopped the pantothenic acid, and after a couple of months, the pain got worse again. He has now started the vitamin again, again he feels better, and this time he intends to continue taking pantothenic acid.

Lois's Hands

Lois is the seventy-three-year-old mother of a friend of mine. Because she had a lot of aches and pains, with those in her hands by far the worst, her son talked her into trying pantothenic acid. He even mailed her a supply of the pills (she is retired and lives two thousand miles away from him).

After a month on pantothenic acid, Lois reported that her hands were much better. She continues to take pantothenic aid.

Judy's Hands

Judy has had pain in her finger joints for about the last nine years, with the number of joints affected and the severity of the pain increasing gradually over that time. Although she has never been formally diagnosed, arthritis seems to run in her family—both her aunt and her grandmother were diagnosed with arthritis (though they weren't told specifically what kind), and her sister, though never formally diagnosed, also has joint pain. For Judy, as for so many other sufferers, the pain is worst when the weather is damp.

Five or six years ago, on my recommendation, she started taking pantothenic acid, and she found that after about a week, her pain was completely gone. During the following years, as long as she remembered to take the vitamin, the pain stayed away; but often, feeling fine, she would forget, and after about a week without pantothenic acid, the pain would come back. As you might guess, she would then restart the vitamin, and again the pain would go away.

What Their Doctors Said

Rosemary, Pat, and Larry told their doctors about their successes with pantothenic acid. Pat reported that her doctor "wasn't the least bit interested," Rosemary's doctor made no special comment, and Larry's doctor was noncommittal, saying only that it was "interesting." None of these doctors showed any desire to find out more about the use of pantothenic acid for joint pain, but at least they didn't tell their patients to stop taking it. (For more on doctors' attitudes towards pantothenic acid, see Chapter Nine.)

The rest of those who tried the vitamin on my recommendation never bothered to tell their doctors at all. All that mattered to them was that they felt much better.

RAISING QUESTIONS

These are some of the success stories. There were, of course, failures—people who tried pantothenic acid and got nothing from it. And the placebo effect definitely reared its head at least once in these informal settings. A man I met on the Internet tried the vitamin and reported vast improvement in his arthritis overnight, with an accompanying boost in his spirits and energy level. But only two weeks later, the improvement, as well as his good spirits and extra energy, had vanished. I hadn't told him that, judging from the people who had tried it before and from the scientific research, the vitamin was likely to take at least a week, maybe more, to do anything; I had just suggested that he try it for a while and see what happened. I wasn't surprised, then, when the effects he was so happy about had vanished. I think they were entirely in his mind, a classic case of the placebo effect. At that point, he told me he was giving up on pantothenic acid, and I assumed that I would never hear from him again. But I did, a few weeks later, when he let me know that he had tried some other substance recommended by someone (I can't remember what it was), and his arthritis, his spirits, and his energy had once again improved immediately. I haven't heard from him since.

It's interesting that some of the people who benefited had old injuries in their arthritic joints, but others didn't. And some people found some joints improved and other joints did not. Another man I found on the Internet tried the vitamin and reported that although his joints above the waist were much better, with significant pain reduction and greatly increased mobility, his arthritic hip was still very bad.

How to judge who might be helped and who might not? Only more research can answer that question. But, though arthritis research continues on many fronts these days (in the past year, I've gotten two requests in the mail from the Arthritis Foundation of Illinois for donations to help find the causes and cures for arthritis), it isn't paying any attention to pantothenic acid. How to change that? My decision to write this book was part of the attempt. And the other part involved my co-author, Dr. Scheiner.

Judy, whose hands improved so much, is Dr. Scheiner's wife. It was her reaction to the vitamin, as much as anything else, that convinced him there was a real effect taking place. And that led to our running our own study of the effects of pantothenic acid on arthritis, which we'll take a look at now.

OUR OWN RESEARCH

When I decided to write a book about arthritis and pantothenic acid, I knew that I didn't know much about either subject. So I began to prowl one of the local medical school libraries, reading journals and handbooks, following up footnotes and searching through indexes. I also began to talk about the book to any biological scientist or doctor friend who was willing to listen. (You can find the names of some of these amazingly patient people in the Acknowledgments.)

One of them was Dr. Samuel M. Scheiner, who, at that time, was teaching biology and statistics at Northern Illinois University. As noted earlier in this chapter, his wife Judy had great success in using pantothenic acid for her own joint pain. And one day, as we were chatting about the planned book, and about how little scientific research I had been able to locate in this area, he said, "You know, you could run your own study. It wouldn't cost a lot to do a small one."

The idea intrigued me, and over the next couple of months I thought about it more and more. I had never done any scientific research of my own, though in college I had either observed or helped around the edges of a couple of biological research projects (courtesy of boyfriends and roommates). I had also been reading about other people's research in magazines like *Scientific American* for most of my adult life. The more I thought about it, the more interesting the whole concept of doing some research of my own became. Dr. Scheiner, who was an experienced researcher, would design the study, I would recruit volunteers and gather all the data, and he would analyze the numbers and come out with a conclusion.

The Study

We agreed to give it a try. Dr. Scheiner drew up an Informed Consent Form, and under his direction I worked out the General Instructions, the Questionnaire, and the Chart. The Informed Consent Form is a requisite for all research done on human beings. The Questionnaire was intended to provide some basic information about the subject that would help us analyze the results. The Chart enabled the subject to keep track of his or her pain and stiffness for the duration of the study. (All of these forms are shown in the Appendix.)

The plan was to persuade as many people as possible to record their arthritis symptoms for five weeks, during four of which they would be taking unidentified pills (the first week would be a baseline week, without pills). Some of these pills would be the vitamin and some would be a placebo (not a vitamin at all, just an innocuous pill that looked like the vitamin), but the volunteers would not know which was which. Some volunteers would take the vitamin for two weeks and then the placebo for two weeks. Others would take the placebo for two weeks and then the vitamin. We would compare the effects of the two different kinds of pills with each other and with the baseline week. It seemed simple, except for the analysis of the data, and fortunately, I didn't have to do that part.

For the recruitment drive, I started with my friends, and my friends' friends, and my friends' parents—anyone who had arthritis and didn't already use pantothenic acid. I limited my recruitment to people who only took over-the-counter painkillers and anti-inflammatories (at that time, acetaminophen, aspirin, and ibuprofen); I knew I wouldn't get many volunteers if I told them they couldn't take any pain medication, but at least I could avoid muddying the waters with powerful prescription drugs.

With these limitations, I ran through my personal contacts fairly quickly. Then I turned to the Internet, where I had noticed an on-line arthritis support group. There, and in other science and medicine-oriented Internet groups, I posted requests for volunteers who had either osteoarthritis or rheumatoid arthritis, which we had finally settled on as our areas of investigation.

There were a lot of inquiries. Some people didn't qualify because of the medications they were taking. Others were understandably reluctant to swallow mystery pills provided by a total stranger. Others just wanted to know what we were testing so that they could go ahead and take it on their own. Eventually, though, eighty-three people volunteered, of whom sixty-four actually returned their signed Informed Consent Forms and were sent charts, instructions, and containers of mystery pills. Fifty-seven of these people had rheumatoid arthritis or osteoarthritis (the others were leftovers from the time before we had decided to focus on these two kinds). Of those, twenty-three never returned their charts, and four messed theirs up to the point of unusability. That left thirty people who completed the study, a little more than a third of the original volunteers.

Human beings, I had discovered, were a lot harder to do research on than rats. Rats, after all, are stuck in their cages and can't walk away. Still, Dr. Scheiner said that for a preliminary study, which was all we could do, given our limited funds, thirty subjects was good enough.

I turned the data over to him for analysis. I had only a vague idea of what I was looking at when I scanned the charts; my last college course in statistics was more than thirty years in the past, and I didn't do all that well in it. Still, even I could see that some people, at least, had done better on pantothenic acid than on the placebo.

Even so, I was surprised at the results. The subjects with osteoarthritis had gotten nothing from the vitamin. But those with rheumatoid arthritis had gotten significant results. They had improved while on pantothenic acid. Some had improved more and some less, but across the whole group, the pain and stiffness in their joints (as reported on their daily Charts) had definitely diminished, and that had not happened on the placebo. (For Dr. Scheiner's more detailed description of the study, see the Appendix.)

What did this mean? Was Dr. Annand wrong? Did his osteoarthritic patients just experience the placebo effect? Or will further research show that, for whatever reason, some people with osteoarthritis do improve on pantothenic acid? We don't know. The large scale studies that would answer those questions just haven't been done.

And we're left with other questions, too. Rheumatoid

arthritis looks like it responds to pantothenic acid, both in our own study and previous ones. Can other researchers confirm these results? Will other forms of arthritis respond, too, especially other forms of inflammatory arthritis? What about tendinitis, bursitis, and the rest? Most of the people you read about in the beginning of this chapter, who tried pantothenic acid informally and found relief from their pain, did not know what kind of arthritis they had. Either their doctors hadn't told them or they had never been formally diagnosed; they just knew they had pain. Some had arthritis as a result of old injuries, which are usually considered to be sources of osteoarthritis (Mark's was actually diagnosed as that). Yet only Annand's study showed pantothenic acid helping osteoarthritis. Again, more research is called for. (In Chapter Ten, we'll talk about why it hasn't been done.)

WHAT DOES THIS ALL MEAN FOR YOU?

Pantothenic acid has worked for some people, and it may work for you. In the next chapter we'll talk about appropriate dosages of the vitamin, which seem to be a highly individual matter. And since we spent so much time in Chapter Three talking about the bad side effects of so many of the standard arthritis treatments, we'll talk about the safety of pantothenic acid.

Chapter 8

SAFETY AND DOSAGES

Pantothenic acid may be the safest vitamin of them all. In very large doses, many other vitamins can be toxic. Vitamins A and D, for example, can be quite dangerous in high dosages. Because both are oil soluble and not eliminated in the urine, they stay in the body for a long time, stored in the liver, where they can build up to harmful levels.

Over a period of months, 75,000 to 500,000 International Units of vitamin A (retinol) per day can lead to nausea, loss of hair, drying and scaling of the skin, fatigue, blurred vision, headache, bone damage, enlargement of the liver, and even cirrhosis. Arctic explorers have been known to experience the symptoms of vitamin A overdose after eating polar bear liver, which stores extremely large amounts of the vitamin (polar bears, though, don't seem to have any trouble with those amounts). Outside of such special circumstances, our diets don't contain such high levels of this vitamin, but we can achieve them by taking too many supplements. One can easily buy vitamin A in 25,000 I.U. capsules at drug stores and health food stores, and it would only take three of those capsules a day to reach the level of overdose. The instructions on the bottles, of course, normally say to take one capsule a day, but inevitably some people think that if one is good, three must be better. This is dangerous reasoning when it comes to some vitamins.

Beta-carotene, on the other hand, the substance that our own bodies transform into vitamin A as needed, is not toxic, and some supplements now contain it in preference to, or in addition to, vitamin A itself. Very large doses of beta-carotene will, however, make your skin turn yellowish. This can also be achieved if you eat a *lot* of carrots (a good natural source of beta-carotene).

Vitamin D overdose, which occurs at a level of 50,000 to 100,000 International Units per day in adults (2,000 to 4,000 I.U. in infants), is harder to achieve because our diets tend to be fairly low in vitamin D, and even supplements generally contain far lower levels (in the range of 400 I.U.) of the vitamin. If you were to overdose, though, the symptoms would include weakness, fatigue, loss of appetite, nausea, vomiting, and eventually kidney damage.

The water-soluble vitamins, in general, are much less dangerous because they are eliminated from the body in the urine relatively quickly. Even so, megadoses of niacin (more than 1,000 to 2,000 mg per day) may cause irregular heart beat and liver damage, and megadoses of vitamin B_6 (more than 500 mg daily for more than two months) can cause bone pain and muscle weakness, as well as numbness, and other nerve disorders. Even vitamin C, which is considered safe in very large doses, has its drawbacks—in doses of more than 500 mg per day, it may cause diarrhea. If you are thinking about taking very large doses of any vitamins, you should read about them first.

Which is what I did for pantothenic acid. And I found that its complete safety in human beings is well established (Fox 1984; Heiby 1988; Marks 1989; *FDA Consumer* 1989).

Human beings have taken as much as 10,000 mg and even 15,000 mg a day for as long as nineteen months without any ill effects. This is a huge megadose of pantothenic acid, compared to the Daily Value/RDA of a mere 10 mg.

DOSAGES

As we've said elsewhere in this book, we are all different. The amount of pantothenic acid that works for one person may not work for another. For yet another person, the vitamin may not work at all, in any dosage. And some people may find that at different times in their lives, they need different amounts. I'm one of those, and we'll look at my dosage shortly. First, let's take another look at the animal studies and see what we can learn from them.

Animal Studies

In the wound-healing experiments, the doctors in Strasbourg found that rabbits given a supplement of 20 mg/kg per day of injected pantothenic acid (in addition to their ordinary laboratory animal diet) healed faster and better than rabbits not given any extra pantothenic acid. That's 20 mg of pantothenic acid per kilogram of body weight per day (a kilogram is 1,000 g or a million mg). Rabbits are fairly small creatures, and these particular rabbits weighed about 2.5 kg each (about 5.5 pounds), so their pantothenic acid dosage was about 50 mg per day. The proportional amount a 150-pound (68 kg) human being would take would be 1,360 mg of pantothenic acid per day.

In the adjuvant arthritis experiments done in Belarus, the rats were given 30 mg/kg per day of pantothenic acid. This translates to 2,040 mg for a 150-pound human being.

In the longevity experiments done on mice by Drs. Williams and Pelton, the mice were given about 300 mcg per day of pantothenic acid each in their drinking water. With a typical laboratory mouse weighing in at about 30 g, this would be 100 mg/kg of body weight or, in human terms, 6,800 mg for a 150-pound person.

But these were animal studies, and animal dosages don't necessarily translate neatly into human dosages. And we are, of course, interested in human dosages.

How Much Should You Take?

In the experiments on skin inflammation done in the former Soviet Union, human subjects showed good results (the inflammation cleared up) with 1,000 mg of pantothenic acid per day.

In the studies on exercise, the athletes showed increased endurance while taking 2,000 mg per day.

In the study of the skin inflammation of lupus, subjects took anywhere from 5,000 to 15,000 mg per day. They also took 1,000 to 2,000 mg of vitamin E per day, equivalent to about 1,500 to 3,000 I.U.

J.C. Annand gave his osteoarthritis patients pills totalling 25 mg per day, with good results.

Barton-Wright and Elliot gave their subjects with rheumatoid arthritis daily injections of 50 mg of pantothenic acid and got good results. They gave their osteoarthritis patients pills totalling 100 mg of pantothenic acid and 60 mg of cysteine per day and also got good results.

The General Practitioner Group administered an escalating series of pills to their patients: 500 mg a day for the first two days, then 1,000 mg a day for three days, then 1,500 mg a day for four days, and then 2,000 mg a day for the remainder of the eight-week test period. (Presumably, they were easing their patients into use of the vitamin, to avoid some sort of shock to their systems.) They got good results for those of their patients who had rheumatoid arthritis.

That's a broad range of dosages. Can we narrow it down a little?

When I started taking pantothenic acid, I thought I needed to spread my pills out through the day in order to keep a high level of the vitamin in my blood. This was what I understood from Adelle Davis's book, and it certainly worked. While the pain was bad, I took 200 mg of the vitamin six times a day, for a total of 1,200 mg. Later experimentation showed me that I could drop down to 200 mg a day, in a single dose, for long-term maintenance. That lasted for almost fifteen years, until a new place—my knee (site of an old injury)—started to hurt. Then, by gradually increasing my pantothenic acid dosage, two weeks at a time, I discovered my new maintenance dose, 600 mg per day (I verified this by lowering it several times, only to find the pain returning each time). This, too, worked fine as a single dose.

Earlier this year, I started to get twinges in my knee again, especially when the weather was bad. This made me raise my dosage to 1,100 mg per day, which worked nicely. Maybe I'm becoming tolerant of the vitamin and need more now to achieve the same old effect, or maybe it's just my metabolism changing, now that I'm approaching menopause.

Betty, who had pain in her fingers, took 250 mg until the pain went away, and now she is on a maintenance dose of 100 mg a day. Pat, Larry, and Rosemary take 500 mg a day. Dave, Mark, and Lois take 1,000 mg a day. Dr. Scheiner and I tested our osteoarthritis and rheumatoid arthritis volunteers with 500 mg per day.

The real answer to how much pantothenic acid to take is that everyone has to find his or her own proper level. I used to recommend 500 mg a day when that was approximately what I was taking. Now I suggest starting with 1,000 mg and, if it has an effect (after you've given it a month or so to do something), lowering the dose by 200 or 250 mg every two weeks until you find your own best level. (These happen to be two of the sizes pantothenic acid pills come in.) Dosage may be weight related (Dave, for example, is a very big guy, almost twice Larry's weight); certainly, some of the animal researchers thought it must be. It may also be related to the severity of the arthritis. Since you can't overdose at the levels I'm suggesting, you won't be doing yourself any harm if you're taking too much. But of course, there's no point in wasting pills and money by taking more than you need.

And do take pantothenic acid with meals. Vitamins work with food, so give yours some fuel.

HOW TO FIND PANTOTHENIC ACID

Like other vitamins, pantothenic acid is not a prescription drug. You can buy it over the counter. You can find it at most places that sell a broad array of individual vitamins. It will usually be shelved with the other seven B vitamins: B_1 (thiamine), B_2 (riboflavin), B_6 (either pyridoxine, pyridoxal, or pyradoxamine—all three forms show the vitamin activity), B_{12} (cyanocobalamine), B_3 (niacin, also known as nicotinic acid; its relative niacinamide also shows the vitamin activity and is often substituted for it), folic acid (also known as folate or folacin), and biotin. Walgreen Drug Stores, Osco Drug, and Kmart often carry pantothenic acid (but not always). General Nutrition Centers (GNC) and other large health food stores should have it. With a little hunting, you can probably find sources near you. Try the telephone directory listings for "Vitamins & Food Supplements—Retail" or "Health & Diet Food Products—Retail."

Although pantothenic acid is vitamin B_5, you won't often find it called by its number. (To make matters more confusing, scientists in the former Soviet Union call it vitamin B_3.) Instead, the front of the label on this particular vitamin bottle will generally just say "pantothenic acid," and the small print on the back will say "calcium pantothenate," or "D-calcium pantothenate," or "calcium d-pantothenate."

Pantothenic acid, sodium pantothenate, calcium pantothenate, and panthenol are all forms of the vitamin. (Just as ascorbic acid, sodium ascorbate, and calcium ascorbate are all forms of vitamin C.) Calcium pantothenate is the standard commercially produced version. Chemically speaking, it is a white crystalline salt, though not the kind of salt you sprinkle on your food (sodium chloride), since it contains neither sodium nor chloride. In this form it is not an acid, and it won't eat away at your stomach lining. And, it is not the kind of salt that may have an effect on blood pressure or fluid retention, so if you're on a low-sodium or low-salt diet, you can take pantothenic acid without worrying. As an additive to breakfast cereal, it is usually just called "pantothenate."

Pantothenic acid comes in tablets and capsules of various sizes, including 100 mg, 200 mg, 250 mg, 500 mg, and 1,000 mg. It is also found in "B-50," "B Complex 50," "B-100," and "B Complex 100" tablets or capsules, which contain either 50 or 100 mg each of most of the major B vitamins, pantothenic acid included (although they usually have much smaller amounts of B_{12}, folic acid, and biotin). We do not recommend taking more than one or two of these group vitamins per day without doing some reading on the overdose levels of all those other B vitamins first. You should not depend solely on such group vitamins for your high dose of pantothenic acid.

Many vitamin manufacturers offer pantothenic acid by itself under such brand names as KAL, Thompson, TwinLab, Solgar, GNC, and a host of others. A large health food store may carry several different brands and many different strengths. Prices vary by both brand and strength but are quite reasonable. A hundred tablets of the 250 mg size might cost seven dollars. A hundred capsules of the 500 mg size could run eleven dollars. (Yes, the larger sizes are more economical, as with breakfast cereal and laundry detergent.) At these prices, 1,000 mg per day would cost 22 to 28 cents, and a month's supply of pantothenic acid would run between $6.60 and $8.40. That's comparable to what you might spend on ibuprofen.

It's out there, it's safe, it's not expensive, and it doesn't require a prescription. It's worth trying. If you'd feel better talking to your doctor about it before taking it, by all means do so. But be prepared for his reaction. (We'll talk about that in the next chapter.)

Chapter 9

You and Your Doctor

Doctors know some things about vitamins. They study the biochemistry of vitamins in medical school, and they also learn a little about nutrition. They are aware of the various recognized deficiency diseases—scurvy (vitamin C deficiency), rickets (vitamin D deficiency), beriberi (vitamin B_1 deficiency), and pellagra (niacin deficiency). They know that a lack of vitamin A can cause night blindness (the inability to see at night or in dim light) and a lack of vitamin B_{12} can cause pernicious anemia (where the bone marrow doesn't make enough red blood cells for the body's needs).They know about folic acid deficiency now, since it's been in the news prominently lately as a likely cause of spina bifida and cleft palate in the babies of women who don't get enough of that vitamin during pregnancy. And they are becoming increasingly aware of the mounting evidence for the beneficial effects—the reduction of the risk of heart disease and cancer—of large doses of beta-carotene and vitamins C and E. (My ophthalmologist, with whom I often discuss vitamins, started taking them a couple of years ago.)

But ask your doctor what pantothenic acid is, and chances are he won't even recognize the name.

Part of the reason for this is, of course, that pantothenic acid doesn't have some well-known deficiency disease associated with it. Nor has research shown it to have an effect on heart disease or cancer, diseases with high profiles and potentially lethal outcomes. Pantothenic acid is just a quiet little vitamin, near the bottom of the list on most multi-vitamin supplement labels, not even added to most foods that are enriched with other B vitamins. Easy to forget about.

So you'll probably have to explain that it's a vitamin. And at that point, unless you have an unusual doctor, he or she is not likely to have a positive attitude toward your taking it for your arthritis.

Doctors' attitudes toward vitamin supplements for arthritis tend to fall into two categories: passively negative and actively negative.

THE PASSIVELY NEGATIVE DOCTOR

The passively negative doctor doesn't believe that whatever therapy you want to try will work, but as long as he thinks it won't harm you, he doesn't care if you use it or not. And if you do improve after going on that therapy, he won't attribute your improvement to it. He may dismiss that therapy out of hand; he may not even want to discuss it. Or, he may say that your improvement is a coincidence, due to something else, perhaps even just the passage of time. Or he may attribute it to the placebo effect, which we will discuss a little later.

Pat, Rosemary, and Larry, whose stories of success with pantothenic acid were told in Chapter Seven, all had doctors who were passively negative about the vitamin. Pat's and Rosemary's doctors simply paid no attention to the apparent role of pantothenic acid in their improvement—they would not acknowledge it, they wouldn't even discuss it. And

Larry's doctor only made a noncommittal remark about it, the equivalent of a shrug. By their attitudes, these doctors were rejecting any possibility that pantothenic acid could have an effect on their patients' joint pain. Fortunately, they didn't tell their patients to stop taking it, and this, of course, is the hallmark of the passively negative doctor; he or she just thinks the vitamin is irrelevant.

My own orthopedic surgeon fell into this category. As I said in Chapter One, he gave up on my arthritis and left me with a prescription for codeine and the advice of bed rest, not to mention a bad case of depression. Months later, after I had found that pantothenic acid got rid of my pain and gave me back a normal life, I called him to give a full report on my happy discovery. But he was unimpressed. "It's the placebo effect," he said. And he never would budge from that opinion.

"Placebo" is a Latin word meaning "I shall please," and it refers to the patient's expectation that a treatment will help him. The placebo effect is the human mind saying, "This will work," and the human mind can have a powerful influence on the human body. The placebo effect can show up in scientific research, which is why new medications are tested against pills that contain substances (like plain sugar) known not to have any effect on the ailment in question. Such pills are called placebos. If the medication has a significantly greater effect than the placebo does, then it is doing something real that doesn't depend on the patient's mental attitude. (See Chapter Seven and the Appendix for more on placebos.)

So, my orthopedic surgeon thought pantothenic acid wasn't actually doing anything in and of itself. Its positive effect, he was telling me, was the result of my mind acting on my body. My family doctor, too, who had originally referred me to the orthopedic surgeon, felt the same way. Since the research on pantothenic acid and arthritis is so little known, your own doctor may take this point of view.

Also an aspect of this passively negative attitude, is the automatic assumption that no one who eats a well-balanced diet needs vitamin supplements. If you're not obviously suffering from scurvy, beriberi, or pellagra (and few of us are, these days), you must be getting enough vitamins. The FDA says so. So why waste your money on supplements?

THE ACTIVELY NEGATIVE DOCTOR

Your doctor may also take a more serious approach to the use of pantothenic acid. As we saw in Chapter Eight, it is possible to overdose on some vitamins, and the consequences can be grave. Without knowing a great deal about pantothenic acid, your doctor may assume that it, too, is dangerous in large doses. Or, he or she may simply accept the opinion of the Arthritis Foundation on the use of vitamins for arthritis.

The Arthritis Foundation, which is a nationwide organization with local chapters in many states, is the major fundraiser for arthritis research in the United States. (You may have seen its line of arthritis pain-relievers at your drugstore, or ads for them on TV—they are one way the Arthritis Foundation raises money.) This organization is responsible for many publications, including the exhaustive and technical *Primer on the Rheumatic Diseases*, which is essentially an entire medical school course on these diseases and intended for doctors. It also publishes dozens of brochures for arthritis sufferers, on every aspect of arthritis from ankylosing spondylitis to systemic lupus erythematosus, and from exercise to coping with stress.

One of these brochures, "Arthritis—Unproven Remedies," lists a number of things people do for their arthritis that the Arthritis Foundation considers harmless and others it considers harmful. On the "harmless" list, among other remedies, are copper bracelets and acupuncture, both of which have shown some evidence of benefit to arthritis sufferers, but which do need further research for confirmation. Thus, they are "unproven." On the "harmful" list are such remedies as DMSO (dimethyl sulfoxide), drugs with hidden ingredients like steroids, and large doses of vitamins. DMSO, an industrial solvent, is usually applied to the skin over a painful joint, and it can have an anti-inflammatory effect on that joint. But it is dangerous to use because it sinks right through the skin so effectively that it can take other substances with it, for example the dye in your clothing. Clothing dye is not something you want inside your body, and so DMSO seems to belong on that "harmful" list. As for steroids, especially when you don't know you're taking them, they have significant dangers (see Chapter Three for more on steroids). American patients who have visited certain clinics in Mexico for DMSO treatments have actually been given other drugs instead, without their knowledge, including steroids and powerful NSAIDs (Panush 1993). (See Chapter Three for more on steroids and NSAIDs.) And, as we noted in Chapter Eight, large doses of some vitamins can be dangerous. So the Arthritis Foundation, which is an authority in this arena, makes sense on all these counts. Why shouldn't your doctor assume its opinion applies equally to the vitamin pantothenic acid?

The Arthritis Foundation's other argument, which your doctor may also agree with, is that taking vitamins may keep you from using real medication—that is, prescription medication that has been proved to alleviate the inflammation of arthritis and stave off its destructive effects.

YOUR BEST APPROACHES

You can counter all of these arguments.

You can tell your doctor that eating a well-balanced diet does not guarantee that you will take in even the RDA/Daily Value of pantothenic acid. As we saw in Chapter Five, the processing and cooking of food can lower its pantothenic acid content so much that an average day's meals—even generous meals—cannot reach the FDA's recommended allotment. You can show your doctor Chapter Five, especially the tables that list the very small amounts of pantothenic acid found in various foods and various meals (Tables 5.1, 5.6, 5.8, and 5.9). You can compare your own average daily intake to these tables and argue that, based on the FDA's own Daily Values, at least some supplementation would be good for you.

You can point out that this vitamin, unlike some others, is not harmful even in doses ten, fifteen, or even twenty times higher than the ones you would be taking. And people have taken those ultra-high levels for as long as nineteen months at a stretch without any negative side effects. Arthritis sufferers have taken pantothenic acid for many years at the lower levels that you will be using, at least one of them (me) for twenty-five years, without any trouble. The vitamin handbooks that can be found in any medical school library also agree that large doses of pantothenic acid won't hurt you.

There is also no evidence that pantothenic acid interferes with the action of any medication (or any other vitamin). So you should be able to continue taking your NSAIDs, your steroid, or your SAARDs while using it. One group of lupus patients took massive doses of pantothenic acid and vitamin E while also being treated with steroids, and there were no problems with the combination (Welsh 1954).

As for not taking your real medication—most doctors would be happy to wean you off of those drugs because of their dangers. An orthopedic surgeon I met a couple of years ago (socially, not as a patient) was trying to do just that—switch his arthritis patients from NSAIDs to acetaminophen—because of the NSAIDs' side effects.

The placebo effect is the toughest argument to fight. To counter that argument, you can ask your doctor to read this book, especially Chapters Six, Seven, and the Appendix, which all deal with the scientific research done on pantothenic acid and arthritis over the last thirty-five years. Or he or she can read the original scientific articles, which are listed at the back of this book in the Bibliography for Chapter Six.

But after your doctor reads all of this, he or she might still be unconvinced. The limited amount of research that has been done on pantothenic acid and arthritis is promising, but it isn't definitive. For that, much more research is necessary; large numbers of people must be tested, statistics must be gathered. So your doctor might say that, while interesting, none of this proves that pantothenic acid will actually work on you. At this point, you should argue that while it may not prove anything, it certainly does suggest that pantothenic acid is worth trying.

When I told my gynecologist about my experience with pantothenic acid and about my orthopedic surgeon's reaction, he said, "What do you care if it's a placebo effect? If it works for you, take it."

So, if your doctor is still doubtful after all you've told him, fall back on the ultimate argument—ask him or her to humor you, to bear with your harmless little foibles and see what happens. You will know whether or not pantothenic acid works for you, no matter what your doctor says, and what's important is how you feel, isn't it?

TAKING NOTICE

As with any new therapy, working with your doctor, or getting your doctor to work with you, is important. If enough doctors carefully monitor the progress that their arthritis patients make with pantothenic acid, word will spread about the vitamin's usefulness. Formal research articles are not the only way for an experimental therapy to attract attention; published letters in medical journals can do it also. J.C. Annand (mentioned in Chapter Six) reported his own research in "Letters to the Editors" columns in two British medical journals. Doctors also communicate with each other personally at medical conferences and through local medical societies. If they hear about it often enough, doctors who are skeptical about the use of vitamins for arthritis may begin to take another look at pantothenic acid and to give it serious consideration as a legitimate therapy for some people.

The study of the effect of pantothenic acid on patients with osteoarthritis and rheumatoid arthritis done by the General Practitioner Research Group was a project undertaken by a group of practicing physicians, not by scientists working for a drug company or a university. They were just a bunch of doctors who happened to notice the earlier research and agreed among themselves to try that new therapy on some of their patients (and a placebo on others). They were willing to put in the time and effort required to monitor those patients closely for two months and then to analyze the results. If more of this kind of small-scale research can be done, the medical community can be convinced that something real is going on, that pantothenic acid may well have an important place in the arsenal of weapons against arthritis. Then someone, somewhere, may be encouraged to do the necessary large-scale, double-blind studies required to prove statistically that the successful use of pantothenic acid is not a placebo effect. Such studies would also determine which kinds of arthritis can be helped by pantothenic acid and which cannot, and what the proper dosages are.

In a small but important way, you can help all of this along. This chapter has been about dealing with your doctor's likely negative attitudes toward using pantothenic acid for your arthritis. Talking to your doctor about alternative treatments for arthritis can be an uncomfortable and even embarrassing experience. For some people, it is simpler to just use the stuff and not mention it to the doctor. Certainly, several of my friends who use pantothenic acid successfully have never told their doctors about it. Many of them just don't want the bother of dealing with the doctor about their arthritis yet again—they've gone through so many medications and they've been so unsatisfied with them that they are just happy to be feeling better. They check off arthritis as being something they don't have to complain to their doctors about anymore.

But if we don't tell our doctors about the substances that alleviate our pain and let us get on with reasonably normal lives again, they'll never know why we didn't come back for another prescription for some powerful NSAID. They'll certainly never know that we didn't buy that next bottle of ibuprofen. So, if pantothenic acid helps you, tell your doctor, or at least write him or her a letter. Share the information, and add your small piece to the evidence in favor of large-scale research. Persuading doctors to pay attention to pantothenic acid as a legitimate therapy for inflammatory arthritis may be a long, slow process. But the ultimate outcome could be a lot less suffering for a lot of people.

It would be much simpler, of course, if we could point to some big research study on pantothenic acid and arthritis, preferably published in some major medical journal, and say, "See what we mean?" But we can't, and in the next chapter, we'll take a look at the reasons why that study has not been done yet.

Chapter 10

THE FUTURE

When my husband suggested that I start this book project, I told him that I would do it only if I could find some real scientific research to back up the use of pantothenic acid for arthritis. As we saw in Chapter Six, that research does exist, though there is not a lot of it, and there has not been any done in the English-speaking world (aside from Dr. Scheiner's and my study) since the General Practitioner Group published their work in 1980.

Why has there been so little research on a treatment for arthritis that has shown such promise? One would think that there would be follow-up, at the very least, for rheumatoid arthritis, which gave the clearest and most positive results. One would also think that other forms of arthritis, especially the other kinds of inflammatory arthritis, would be looked at. The evidence for pantothenic acid's effect on inflammation, particularly the research done in the former Soviet Union, certainly seems pretty solid. Why has the pantothenic acid-arthritis connection been ignored?

There are a lot of answers to that question. First, there is the barrier of conservatism. For a long time, the prevailing wisdom has been that anyone who eats a well-balanced diet doesn't need vitamins. The medical community has a longstanding prejudice against the use of vitamins to treat any disease except a few recognized deficiency diseases, like scurvy, beriberi, and pellagra. Doctors may have prescribed multivitamins for their pregnant patients, just to be sure that mothers-to-be and their developing babies get enough—after all, pregnancy is a time of extra nutritional demands—but those doses are low, just in the range of the RDA/Daily Value. Large doses of vitamins have generally been dismissed as useless. (A good example of this is the controversy a few years back over the use of megadoses of vitamin C for the common cold.) Only recently has this particular barrier begun to come down, as research has demonstrated that large doses of certain vitamins, including beta-carotene (which our bodies turn into vitamin A), C, E, and possibly even folic acid, may well offer protection against cataracts, heart disease, and many forms of cancer.

Still, conservatism abounds. The Arthritis Foundation lists vitamins in large doses as potentially harmful unproven remedies. This does not encourage further research in this area, especially since the Arthritis Foundation funds so much arthritis research.

Another answer to our question about the lack of research is that much of the investigation of the anti-inflammatory properties of pantothenic acid has been published in languages other than English. Szorady's research, for example, was published in German, and Otrokov's in Russian. Dr. Andrej Moiseenok has been doing research on numerous aspects of pantothenic acid for thirty years, but only two articles by him have ever appeared in English-language journals; the rest were in Russian journals. Since very little research these days is published in anything other than English, regardless of what country the researchers live in, scientists simply tend to ignore non-English publications.

Additionally, scientists of the Western world look upon research done in the former Soviet Union as suspect. This is at least partly a result of the Soviet Union's past scientific reputation. From the 1930s to the 1960s, the biological sciences in the Soviet Union were dominated by politically powerful people whose fundamental scientific assumptions (for instance, that changes in an individual living creature that are caused by its environment can be passed on to its descendents) were considered, by the rest of the world's scientists, to have been long ago completely disproved. Research done there was seen by outsiders as politically motivated, scientifically unreliable, even ridiculous, so it was mostly ignored by scientists outside the Soviet Union.

A new generation of scientists has grown up since then, but the prejudice lingers. Some of this is due, not just to the questionable past of Soviet science, but to the fact that articles by researchers in the former Soviet Union are often not well written, which makes their methods and results hard to judge. Perhaps in years to come, as there is more contact between scientists from the West and those in the former Soviet Union, as they communicate over the Internet, and as they have more opportunities to work in each other's countries and to observe each other's research, this situation will change.

In the meantime, even finding non-English language scientific publications is difficult, as I know from my own experience. I had to get my own copy of a 1977 Soviet symposium on pantothenic acid directly from the former Soviet Union. It is not surprising, therefore, that none of the Russian-language articles from that symposium were referred to in the General Practitioner Group study, even though the symposium was published three years before their study was. They may have ignored it, but more likely they just never saw it.

In fact, considering all the journals that are published in English—all the dozens of journals that could bear on the uses of pantothenic acid—it's obvious that even keeping up with them is impossible. (You have no idea how many scientific journals there are until you visit a medical school library!) And in the days before computerized databases, locating an article published in the past required a researcher to page through many reference volumes, each of them the size of the Chicago telephone directory, with print just as small. Even though the articles were organized by subject matter, this was a tedious, frustrating, and eye-straining process. Only in recent years have computerized databases made this process relatively easy. So it isn't surprising that the General Practitioner Group also never saw either the Haslock (1971) article or the second Barton-Wright article (1967) on pantothenic acid and osteoarthritis, even though both were published in English.

All right, we've seen some of the reasons why some of this research is so little known in the English-speaking medical world. But what about the original research done in Great Britain? After all, Barton-Wright and Elliot published their work in *Lancet*, one of the most highly-respected medical journals in the world. What happened after that?

After Barton-Wright and Elliot did their research, Dr. Barton-Wright wrote two short books, *Arthritis: A Deficiency Disease* (London: United Trade Press, 1971) and *Arthritis: Its Cause and Control* (London: Roberts Publications, 1974). Both books are long out of print, and their publishers are no longer in business. Some English friends of mine tracked down the companies that had bought those publishers, but these successor companies had no copies of the books; in fact, they had never heard of them. The giant database at the Chicago Public Library, which lists millions of books in libraries around the world, showed no copies of the first book and only two copies of the second. But when a friend went to the British Library to find one of those two copies, it was no longer in the collection—probably stolen. There may only be one copy in the world, in the Cambridge

University Library, if that one hasn't been stolen, too. So Barton-Wright's books are gone. And Barton-Wright and Elliott are gone, too. Barton-Wright died in 1975, and Elliott was retired by 1977 and died sometime between 1978 and 1981. Without them, the research passed into the hands of the General Practitioner Group. In their article, they called for more research. But they didn't do it, and there matters have stood.

Why? You would think such research would be relatively simple. Round up a bunch of people with arthritis, feed them pills, see how they do. Dr. Scheiner and I did it. Nearly every week, I hear a call on one of our local radio stations for volunteers to test a drug for some big medical research project—most recently, it was hormone replacement for postmenopausal women. Why doesn't someone do a major research project on pantothenic acid and arthritis?

Barton-Wright himself said more scientifically controlled experimental trials were needed. And he also said they would be expensive. Our own small-scale study cost almost four hundred dollars for materials and postage; our time was thrown in for free. Doing anything larger would require money to finance advertising for volunteers, as well as to pay workers to sort, label, and pack the vitamins. In scientific research, such money is provided by grants from government or private institutions, and there is tremendous competition these days for such grants.

And the longer the followup research is delayed, the more common becomes the attitude of "Well, if there were something to it, somebody would be working on it by now" among the public, the scientists, and the agencies giving out grant money.

Perhaps the most important single reason why there has not been any research in the U.S. on pantothenic acid as a treatment for arthritis is that no pharmaceutical company can make any substantial profit from a vitamin. Pharmaceutical companies spend a great deal of money developing new drugs, and they have to make that research investment back and earn a profit for their stockholders on top of it. They do that by patenting their name-brand drugs and charging high prices for them. But no one can patent a vitamin, and no one can charge high prices for them because they are already so widely available and so inexpensive. So there's no reason for any pharmaceutical company to pay for any research on pantothenic acid. That leaves the government as the only potential sponsor for such research: presumably either the National Institute of Arthritis and Musculoskeletal and Skin Diseases, or the Office of Alternative Medicine (both divisions of the National Institutes of Health).

But someone, some scientist, has to want to do that research. Someone has to want to go through all the red tape, all the filling out of forms and writing of proposals, that applying for a government grant involves. Perhaps someone reading this book will take on that challenge. I hope so. This research needs someone who is willing to make a large and long-term commitment to it.

In the past, traditional medicine focused on creating drugs to treat diseases, but recently it has begun to expand to include nutritional approaches to the underlying causes of disease. This is especially true in the case of the antioxidant vitamins, C, E and beta-carotene. Over the last couple of decades, a number of doctors have also suggested alternative approaches to arthritis, many of them involving nutrition and diet. Mostly, though, they required you to eliminate some food or foods (usually something you liked) from your life, which made these diets hard to stick with.

As I write this chapter, however, a nutritional supplement has become the newest doctor-suggested, widely-publicized, alternative treatment for osteoarthritis (though it apparently has no effect on rheumatoid arthritis). A combination of glucosamine and chondroitin sulfate, both found naturally in connective tissue, is being promoted as a cure for osteoarthritis—a treatment that is actually supposed to rebuild damaged cartilage in the joints. The theory here appears to be that if you supply the materials, your body will put them where they are needed.

Predictably, there is controversy over this, as there has been over every alternative arthritis approach. But one aspect of this particular treatment caught my attention. In Chapter Four, I noted that one of the many things that pantothenic acid does in your body is help manufacture some important components of connective tissue. These components are of supreme importance in cartilage. One of them is chondroitin sulfate, and the other, hyaluronic acid, is made in part from glucosamine. Without pantothenic acid, neither could be formed. Could it be possible that people with osteoarthritis are not taking in enough pantothenic acid to enable their bodies to rebuild their damaged cartilage out of the raw materials available in the food they eat? And, might it be a lack of pantothenic acid that somehow prevents the glucosamine/chondroitin sulfate supplement from having any effect on rheumatoid arthritis? Only further research will determine the answers to these questions.

So, while I wait for large-scale research to be done on pantothenic acid, I continue to take it, as I have for almost a quarter of a century. I continue to lead an active, pain-free life because of it, and to spread the word about it. To you, who read this and have joint pain, I can only say that pantothenic acid is worth trying. If it works for you as it has for me and for the other people whose stories I've told in this book, you'll be glad you spent the small amount of money and time required to find out.

Appendix

SINGLE-BLIND STUDY & RELATED MATERIALS

RELIEF OF ARTHRITIS SYMPTOMS BY CALCIUM PANTOTHENATE

If you were to read a typical, formal scientific paper, you would find it obscure and dull. Ideas would be packaged in nice neat bows with a clear logical line running from front to back. It would seem as if the researchers knew exactly what they would find even before they began.

Of course, this is not how real science works. Often the nice logical justifications for the research presented in a paper's introduction are thought up or discovered long after a research project has begun, or even finished. Because of serendipitous discoveries or laboratory disasters, the original purpose for a research project will sometimes be modified or, occasionally, entirely discarded. We have given you a taste of the real process in Chapter Seven. In this Appendix we present a modified version of our formal research paper that we will be publishing in a peer-reviewed journal. In this version, we attempt to cut through the typical scientific jargon and explain the reasoning behind the choices we made in designing the experiment and analyzing the data. We hope that this presentation will give you a better appreciation for both the powers and limitations of the scientific process. Every day you are faced with a myriad of claims about miracle cures; our book could even be seen as one of them. With this presentation, we hope to empower you in making reasoned decisions about both our claims and others that you might encounter.

Our story starts with the anecdotal evidence on the effectiveness of pantothenic acid that is detailed in Chapters One and Seven. In the Introduction of our formal paper we discuss several previous experiments that showed evidence that pantothenic acid could relieve arthritis symptoms. But, we actually found those studies after we had begun this experiment. So, in the spirit of honesty, we can only use the information that we had at hand in describing how we made our decisions.

We knew that rheumatoid arthritis and osteoarthritis are illnesses that affect 1–2 percent and over 20 percent of the adult population, respectively (Wilder 1993; Brandt et al 1993). As detailed in Chapter Three, current drug treatments consist of non-steroidal anti-inflammatory drugs (NSAIDs), corticosteroids, and slow-acting anti-rheumatic drugs (SAARDs). However, these treatments can have serious side effects (Williams 1993). NSAIDs can produce headaches, dizziness and confusion, gastric irritation, and skin rashes as well as rare complications such as toxic amblyopia (dimness of vision), reversible hepatocellular toxicity (liver trouble), and aseptic meningitis (inflammation of the membrane covering the brain, not caused by infection). Corticosteroids can cause skin thinning, ecchymoses (bruise marks), edema (fluid retention in various organs and tissues), gastric ulcers, opportunistic infections, and adrenal suppression (failure of the adrenal glands to secrete their hormones) as well as a steroid-induced osteopenia (bone loss). SAARDs as a group tend to be toxic.

Thus, based on personal experience, we recognized a need for an effective treatment without serious side effects.

Pantothenic acid seemed to be that treatment based on anecdotal evidence. But, in the world of science and medicine, anecdote will get you only so far. Informal observations are a basic fuel that drives the engine of science. Many scientific discoveries start with casual observations, such as Newton's proverbial apple. What make a scientist successful are the abilities to recognize the worth of such casual observations, and to design formal experiments to turn them into scientific theories.

Methods

We knew three things when we started this experiment. First, while pantothenic acid seemed to work for most people, it failed to work for some. So, we wanted to sort out the causes for the successes and failures. Doing so would both tell us to whom to recommend pantothenic acid, and potentially lead us to a mechanism for its success. Second, we knew that effects of the treatment were almost always felt within a week of starting to take pantothenic acid. Third, we knew that the effects wore off within a few days of stopping the administration of pantothenic acid. This last observation was consistent with our knowledge of pantothenic acid as a water-soluble vitamin.

Based on these pieces of knowledge, we designed a single(patient)-blind within-subject paired-sample design experiment. What does all that jargon mean? Scientific research aims at discovering causal mechanisms. To do so, scientists manipulate the world in a controlled manner to see what will happen; they do an experiment. A cornerstone of experimental methodology is to be able to separate chance occurrence, or random correlation, from true cause and effect. To do so, scientists rely on comparisons between treatments and controls. In the treatment, you try out the cause you are investigating. For drug therapy experiments, this means giving your subjects the drug and seeing how they react. Does the drug cure the disease or relieve the symptoms? In the control, you do everything exactly the same as in the treatment, except for leaving out the crucial cause. For drug therapy experiments, this means giving your subjects a placebo, a fake pill, that is identical in sight, smell and taste to the real pill. That way you can tell which results are due to the drug and which are due to either chance occurrences or to the psychological benefits of pill-taking, the "placebo effect."

A typical drug effectiveness experiment is double-blind. This means that neither the doctor giving the drug nor the subject know what treatment they are receiving. The reasoning behind this design is that doctor or patient expectations could bias the outcome. If the patient knew that he was taking the real drug, he might feel better even if the drug had no real effect. If the doctor knew that a particular subject was taking the real drug, she might act differently towards that person or see an improvement where one did not exist. So the usual procedure is to "blind" both the doctor and subject. Both the real pills and the placebos are placed in identical numbered containers, coded by someone who will not be working directly with the subjects. Only after the data are all gathered is the code revealed.

We were able to get around the necessity for blinding both the doctor and the subject because we had the subjects self-report their reactions. Disease classifications and observations were done by the subjects themselves, and the only decisions by us were to reject subjects based on incomplete data. Such a system makes data collection much easier and cheaper. The limitation is that we could only gather data on subjective reactions. Other types of data such as urine concentrations of pantothenic acid or formal tests of stiffness were not available. These additional types of information are very important for determining the extent of treatment effectiveness and for providing additional knowledge of causal mechanisms. Thus, we knew from the start that our experiment would just be a preliminary study. Our hope is that others will follow up with the larger, more complex and expensive experiments.

That explains the "single(patient)-blind" part of the description; what about "within-subject paired-sample"? In a typical drug effectiveness experiment there are two different sets of subjects. One set gets just the real pills and one set gets just the placebo. The weakness of this type of experiment is that you must overcome natural among-subject variation. As we discuss in Chapters Two and Seven, individuals vary tremendously in their disease severity and reactions to a given drug treatment. Some people may be in constant pain while others may have just intermittent attacks. Some people may have a strong reaction to a drug, others a weak reaction, and others no reaction at all. The scientist is trying to pull the signal, the true effect of the drug, out of this noise of variation. This signal detection is the purview of statistics. We discuss the details of our statistical analysis below. The important point here is that a key to signal detection is a large sample size. The greater the number of subjects that you include in your study, the easier it is to detect a true, but weak, signal.

We knew that we would not have the luxury of a large number of subjects, given our shoestring budget and recruiting methods. So, we had to find a way to strengthen our signal detection abilities. We knew from our anecdotal information that the effects of pantothenic acid, if they were to occur, would be manifest after about one week of taking the vitamin and would disappear rapidly upon cessation of ingestion. We later found that other studies observed these same patterns (Barton-Wright and Elliott 1963; General Practitioner Research Group 1980). Thus, a single individual could be given both the treatment and the placebo. The important result was not the absolute level of pain or stiffness that a person experienced (that would vary greatly among individuals), but whether pain and stiffness decreased for each person. An individual could act as her own control, the "within-subject" part. Our statistical analysis would compare a person's pain and stiffness while taking pantothenic acid with his pain and stiffness while taking the placebo, the "paired-sample" part.

The treatment consisted of commercially available calcium pantothenate (KAL, Inc., Woodland Hills, CA) in a carrier of dicalcium phosphate, cellulose, vegetable stearin, stearic acid, guar gum, and silica, at a dosage of two tablets (a total of 500 mg) daily, taken in a single dose. The placebo consisted of commercially available dolomite (calcium carbonate/magnesium carbonate, Nature Made Nutritional Products, Los Angeles, CA) at a dosage of two tablets (a total of 260 mg calcium, 160 mg magnesium) daily, taken in a single dose. As far as we know, dolomite has no effect on arthritis symptoms. The treatment and placebo tablets were indistinguishable by sight and taste.

Subjects included individuals suffering from either osteoarthritis or rheumatoid arthritis as diagnosed by a physician and reported by the subjects themselves. Only individuals that were not taking any pain or anti-inflammatory medication other than aspirin, acetaminophen, or ibuprofen were included in the study. The final sample included 21 subjects with osteoarthritis (15 female and 6 male) and 9 subjects with rheumatoid arthritis (7 female and 2 male). There were 23 subjects who did not return their reports and 4 subjects who were discarded for improperly filling out their reports. We also ended up discarding individuals with other forms of arthritis because the sample sizes were so small that we could not perform a meaningful analysis. The mean number of years since disease onset was 9.6 (1.6 SE, n=25), for those subjects that reported this statistic. (SE stands for "standard error"—more on this later.)

The subjects themselves made daily records of pain and stiffness, each recorded on a 5-point scale. To establish individual baselines, the subjects recorded observations for seven days prior to receiving any treatment. The experiment consisted of fourteen days of calcium pantothenate and fourteen days of the placebo, with half the subjects randomly receiving the treatment first and half receiving the placebo first. This part of the design was to allow for "order" effects. For example, we may have under-estimated the time that it takes for the effects of pantothenic acid to disappear after a person stops taking it. If so, then subjects that took pantothenic acid first might show decreased pain and stiffness when next taking the placebo. Such randomization of drug order is standard practice in experiments in which a single individual takes both treatments. The dosages were actually given to the subjects in lots of fourteen pills each (one week's supply), so subjects were unaware that they were receiving the same treatment for fourteen days. This part of the design was more a fortuitous result of the logistics of giving out the pills, not something that we originally planned on. But, once we realized that we would dole out the pills in this fashion, the benefits of further "blinding" the subjects became obvious.

The various documents sent to volunteers—the Informed Consent Form (Document A-1), the Questionnaire (Document A-2), the General Instructions (Document A-3), and the Chart (Table A-2)—appear at the end of this Appendix.

Statistical analyses were done as a series of paired-sample t-tests. A t-test is a method for deciding if two averages are more different than you would expect by chance alone. It, and all statistical procedures, work in the same way. Consider the following experiment. Take a hundred slips of paper, put numbers from 1 to 5 on them, and put them in a hat. Now, pick out 10 slips and calculate the average of the numbers; the *mean* in standard statistical terminology. Put the slips back, shake up the hat, draw out another 10 slips, and again calculate the mean. Both sets of slips came from the same pile in the same hat. So, in theory, the two means should be the same. But, by chance alone, the first set might have had a lot of 5's, giving a large mean, and the second set might have had a lot of 1's, giving a small mean. Statisticians have worked out how much variation one would see in the mean just due to this random variation. Given two means, one can calculate the probability that those two means came from the same hat with same set of numbers, or from different hats with different sets of numbers.

Separate analyses were performed for individuals with osteoarthritis and rheumatoid arthritis. Although we suspected that the two types would react differently to the treatment, we could not be sure. For each subject the mean values for pain and stiffness were calculated for the 7-day pretreatment period and the second 7-day period of receiving the treatment or the placebo. One-week averages were used to eliminate day-to-day variation, thus making overall treatment effects more apparent. Only the second 7-day treatment period was used because our anecdotal observations indicated that up to one week was necessary for treatment effects to become apparent. This decision, to just use the second 7-day period, was made a *priori*, that is prior to examination of the data. These types of decisions about data analysis must always be made before you look at the data. Otherwise, you could look at all two weeks' worth of results and just pick those days to include in your analysis that show the effect that you want. This is the scientific equivalent of throwing a dart against the wall and then drawing the target around it.

Preliminary analyses indicated that there were no order effects (that is, it didn't matter whether the subjects took the vitamin first or the placebo first), so final analyses were done without including order. One-tailed paired-sample t-tests were performed comparing within-subject differences between pretreatment, treatment, and placebo periods. One-tailed tests were used because we were testing a directional hypothesis that pantothenic acid would decrease pain and stiffness. That is, we did not care if it increased pain and stiffness, a very unlikely possibility given our anecdotal information and what we knew about pantothenic acid.

Results

Calcium pantothenate caused a decrease in the pain and stiffness reported by subjects with rheumatoid arthritis (Table 1). On average, subjects reported a decrease in 0.51

(0.17 SE) units in reported pain relative to the pretreatment levels and 0.71 (0.40 SE) units relative to the placebo.

The SE, or standard error, is a measure of how accurately we have estimated the true mean. The data are just a sample from a larger "hat" that includes all possible arthritis sufferers that we might have recruited for our experiment. If we could have included all 40 million people, we would know the true extent of the vitamin's effectiveness for these people. The standard error would be 0. Instead, we have a sample, and that sample is subject to random variation. While we estimate that the true decrease was 0.51 units relative to pretreatment level, it might actually be smaller or larger than that. There is a 95 percent chance that the true decrease could be as small as 0.12 or as large as 0.90. We can only speak in probabilities, because rare events sometimes happen. Occasionally you might hit the jackpot at the slot machine, even though the odds are well stacked in favor of the house. In general, the true mean will be within 2 standard errors of the estimated mean 95 percent of the time and within 3 standard errors 99 percent of the time.

In the subjects with rheumatoid arthritis, the decreases were highly statistically significant for the comparison between the treatment and the pretreatment, and marginally statistically significant for the comparison between the treatment and the placebo, despite the very small sample size. Put another way, there is just a 1 percent chance ($P = 0.009$, where P indicates probability) that the pantothenic acid had no effect and that the true decrease was 0. Scientists generally use a 5 percent probability as the threshold below which they consider something unlikely to happen by chance alone. There is nothing magical about 5 percent, it has just come about by historical tradition. That being said, it was not just pulled out of a hat. It represents a reasonable compromise between letting science move forward and skepticism about new theories. With a lower threshold, say 1 percent, we might continually ignore promising new avenues of research because we cannot find a strong enough signal through the noise. With a higher threshold, say 10 percent, we might continually be pursuing will-o-the-wisps that are just chance events and not true causes. Where one sets the threshold for a particular experiment, depends on circumstances. For example, if one is testing a potentially life-saving new drug for a fatal disease, one might use a higher threshold so that you do not ignore any even remote possibilities. On the other hand, if one is testing whether a new pesticide causes cancer, one might use a lower threshold because the consequences of being wrong might be deadly. Most important is to realize that the advance of science does not hinge on a single experiment. Many different experiments are done, each with its possibility of being wrong due to random chance. The totality of the evidence across all experiments, provides the strongest evidence for a particular theory.

The effects on stiffness in subjects with rheumatoid arthritis were smaller, although in the same direction: 0.16 (0.14 SE) units and 0.42 (0.29 SE) units, respectively. The t-test approached statistical significance for the comparison of the treatment and the placebo.

In contrast, for subjects with osteoarthritis, no effects were found on reported pain or stiffness. The only statistically significant comparison was for pain in the comparison of the pretreatment and the placebo; the treatment actually showed greater reported pain than the placebo.

Thus, we conclude that pantothenic acid taken orally decreases pain and possibly stiffness for individuals with rheumatoid arthritis with no evidence for any decrease for individuals with osteoarthritis.

Discussion

Our results confirm previous studies. In these studies, oral ingestion of calcium pantothenate appeared to alleviate the symptoms of osteoarthritis (Annand 1962) and rheumatoid arthritis (General Practitioner Research Group 1980).

Similarly, daily intramuscular injections of calcium pantothenate provided relief from pain for individuals with rheumatoid arthritis, although this relief disappeared upon cessation of the injections (Barton-Wright and Elliott 1963). One study (General Practitioner Research Group 1980), using a somewhat different protocol than ours, compared individuals that took only pantothenic acid or a placebo for eight weeks. They found a significant decrease in reported pain in subjects with rheumatoid arthritis; and while stiffness was reduced, the difference between the treatment and placebo groups was not statistically significant. Again, sample sizes were small (n=12 in the treatment group and n=15 in the placebo group). They found no effect of pantothenic acid on pain and stiffness for individuals with osteoarthritis, similar to our findings. Overall, these results suggest that oral doses of pantothenic acid are an inexpensive palliative for rheumatoid arthritis. We discovered these studies only after we had started our experiment. Such additional studies, however, give us much more confidence that our results are not due to simple chance, but indicate a true effect. This is why replication of experiments is important for the progress of science.

The General Practitioner Research Group study and our results contradict those of one study (Annand 1962) that reported a small benefit for persons with osteoarthritis. These differences have two possible explanations. First, Annand may have come across that rare chance event that made no effect look like an effect. Or, Annand may have done his experiment in such a way as to find a true effect that we overlooked with our protocol. Such contradictory results are usually a spur for more research. If, eventually, all other studies continue to show no effect of pantothenic acid on osteoarthritis, then Annand's study will be relegated to the "chance event" bin.

Individuals with rheumatoid arthritis may either have the disease, or may have aggravated symptoms, because of a dietary deficiency or a metabolic defect that leads to the inability to retain pantothenic acid in their systems. Individuals with rheumatoid arthritis were found to have depressed levels of pantothenic acid in whole blood (Barton-Wright and Elliott 1963) and above normal levels of pantothenic acid in their urine (Kalliomaki et al. 1960). These types of supplementary information are very important for scientists when they decide on whether to accept a new theory. They are additional hypotheses or expectations that should be true if the main theory were true. Again, scientists rely on the totality of the evidence, not just a single study or type of study.

Our results, and the difference in response between persons with osteoarthritis and rheumatoid arthritis, suggest a mechanism of action of pantothenic acid. Pantothenic acid has anti-inflammatory properties (Moiseenok et al. 1981). Likely this is the mode of action of pantothenic acid on rheumatoid arthritis. The reversal of effects upon cessation of taking pantothenic acid is consistent with this hypothesis. We speculate that pantothenic acid may also be useful in the treatment of other diseases that involve inflammation, although such demonstrations await further study. Being able to provide a possible mechanism is another important piece of evidence that scientists use. Scientists are looking for causes. While medicine can often proceed by the black-box approach (drug X in, cure Y out), learning about causal mechanisms allows for the development of much more effective treatments. Also, different causes can give the same effect. By providing a possible causal mechanism for the effects of pantothenic acid, we allow other scientists a better chance to test our theories. Scientists are much more likely to embrace, or at least take an interest in, theories that can be tested in many different ways.

In general, our results strongly suggest that additional, larger studies of the effects of pantothenic acid on rheumatoid arthritis are warranted, especially ones that would include a wider set of outcome measures such as disease activity. This conclusion echoes that made 15 years ago (General Practitioner Research Group 1980).

Table A-1

Reported levels of pain and stiffness, based on a 5-point Likert scale, of subjects with rheumatoid arthritis (n = 9) and oseoarthritis (n = 21) during pretreatment, taking calcium pantothenate for 14 days,and taking a placebo for 14 days. Values are means of a 7-day period.

A. Pain

		Treatment			t-tests			
Type of Arthritis		Pretreatment	Calcium Pantothenate	Placebo		1 vs 2	1 vs 3	2 vs 3
Rheumatoid	Mean	2.76	2.25	2.96	*t*	3.01	-0.61	1.77
	SE	0.07	0.23	0.29	*P*	0.009	0.6	0.058
Osteoarthritis	Mean	2.55	2.42	2.31	*t*	0.86	1.87	-0.87
	SE	0.11	0.14	0.16	*P*	0.2	0.038	0.7

B. Stiffness

		Treatment			t-tests			
Type of Arthritis		Pretreatment	Calcium Pantothenate	Placebo		1 vs 2	1 vs 3	2 vs 3
Rheumatoid	Mean	2.65	2.49	2.91	*t*	1.10	-1.17	1.44
	SE	0.17	0.23	0.20	*P*	0.15	0.14	0.09
Osteoarthritis	Mean	2.37	2.25	2.27	*t*	0.75	0.85	0.09
	SE	0.16	0.17	0.16	*P*	0.2	0.2	0.9

Document A-1 Informed Consent Form

You have volunteered to participate in a study on the effects of vitamins in relieving the symptoms associated with arthritis. Because you are a subject in a scientific study, we must inform you of any potential risks or benefits and any side effects that you might experience.

I. Protocol

In this study each subject will receive, at different times, both the vitamin and the placebo. Thus, you will experience both treatment conditions. This method has the benefit of allowing any effects of the vitamin to be calibrated against each person's normal pain and stiffness levels.

II. Risks and Benefits

We know of no possible risks associated with the substances that you will be taking. Both the vitamin being tested and the placebo are commonly available without prescription. Both substances are water soluble, meaning that they are naturally continuously flushed from the body. No known toxic effects have been found at the doses to be used in this study.

III. Effects Experienced

The purpose of this study is to examine the effects of vitamins in relieving pain and stiffness associated with arthritis. We ask, therefore, that you refrain if possible from taking any medication that may mask the symptoms under study. As a result, you may experience pain and/or stiffness on those days that you are taking the placebo or if the treatment has little or no effect. The effects of the vitamin will last only as long as you are taking the treatment. Thus, these treatments will result in neither any long-term harm nor any long-term benefit to you.

If you understand the above statements, please sign and date the statement below. Keep one copy for your records, and return the other to Phyllis Eisenstein.

I understand the above conditions and likely outcomes to me from participating in this study. I hereby grant my consent to participate.

____ ____________

(Signature) (Date)

____

(Please print name)

Document A-2 Arthritis Study Questionnaire

Subject No. ________

Male ________ Female ________

Year of birth ________

What kind of arthritis do you have?

____ Rheumatoid arthritis

____ Osteoarthritis

____ Other ____________________________

____ Don't know

How long have you had arthritis? ______________________

Have you been told by a doctor that you have arthritis?

Yes ________

No ________

Document A-3 Arthritis Study

General Instructions:

As a participant in this five-week study, you will be taking pills and filling out the enclosed questionnaire and chart.

Do not put your name on either sheet.

Your code number is already on both. To begin, please fill out the brief questionnaire. Then proceed each day as follows:

Week 1: Take no pills. This is the baseline week. Just fill in the chart every evening after dinner, evaluating that day.

(Starting with Week 2, you will begin taking pills. Please take them with your dinner.)

Week 2: Each evening, take two pills from the bag marked "Week 2" and fill in the chart.

Week 3: Each evening, take two pills from the bag marked "Week 3" and fill in the chart.

Week 4: Each evening, take two pills from the bag marked "Week 4" and fill in the chart.

Week 5: Each evening, take two pills from the bag marked "Week 5" and fill in the chart.

When the chart is complete (after day 35), use the enclosed envelope to return it and the questionnaire to Phyllis Eisenstein.

Instructions for the chart:

Each evening, rate your pain and stiffness for the day, on the following scale of 1 to 5. If you took painkillers, rate your pain and stiffness as they were before you took those painkillers.

1 = no pain
2 = minor pain (easily ignored)
3 = moderate pain (interfering slightly with activity)
4 = considerable pain (interfering significantly with activity)
5 = extreme pain (incapacitating)

1 = no stiffness
2 = minor stiffness (easily ignored)
3 = moderate stiffness (interfering slightly with activity)
4 = considerable stiffness (interfering significantly with activity)
5 = extreme stiffness (incapacitating)

If you took any painkiller on this day, please list it by name (either brand name or generic) in the space provided. Don't forget that some cold medicines also have painkillers in them. If you are taking the painkiller for something other than your arthritis, please note that. For example:

Day	**Pain**	**Stiffness**	**Medication**
1	2	3	2 Tylenol—not for arthritis
2	3	3	1 Advil

Table A-2 Arthritis Study Chart

Subject No. ___

	Day	Pain	Stiffness	Medication
Week 1	1	___	___	___
	2	___	___	___
	3	___	___	___
	4	___	___	___
	5	___	___	___
	6	___	___	___
	7	___	___	___
Week 2	8	___	___	___
	9	___	___	___
	10	___	___	___
	11	___	___	___
	12	___	___	___
	13	___	___	___
	14	___	___	___
Week 3	15	___	___	___
	16	___	___	___
	17	___	___	___
	18	___	___	___
	19	___	___	___
	20	___	___	___
	21	___	___	___
Week 4	22	___	___	___
	23	___	___	___
	24	___	___	___
	25	___	___	___
	26	___	___	___
	27	___	___	___
	28	___	___	___
Week 5	29	___	___	___
	30	___	___	___
	31	___	___	___
	32	___	___	___
	33	___	___	___
	34	___	___	___
	35	___	___	___

BIBLIOGRAPHY

Chapter One

Davis, Adelle. *Let's Get Well.* New York: Harcourt Brace Jovanovitch, 1965.

Chapter Two

The Harvard Medical School Health Publications Group. *Arthritis: A Harvard Health Letter Special Report.* Boston: Harvard Medical School Health Publications Group, 1995.

MacConnaill, Michael A. "Joints," *Encyclopaedia Britannica Macropaedia,* v. 10, pp. 252-259. Chicago: Encyclopaedia Britannica, Inc. 1974.

"Osteoarthritis," *Encyclopaedia Britannica Micropaedia,* v. VII, p. 613. Chicago: Encyclopaedia Britannica, Inc. 1974.

"Rheumatoid arthritis," *Encyclopaedia Britannica Micropaedia,* v. VIII, p. 549. Chicago: Encyclopaedia Britannica, Inc. 1974.

Rodman, Gerald P. and Benedek, Thomas G. "Connective Tissue Diseases," *Encyclopaedia Britannica Macropaedia,* v. 5, pp. 17-23. Chicago: Encyclopaedia Britannica, Inc. 1974.

Schumacher, H. Ralph (ed.). *Primer on the Rheumatic Diseases, 10th Edition.* Atlanta: Arthritis Foundation, 1993.

Searles, Robert. "Arthritis," *McGraw-Hill Concise Encyclopedia of Science and Technology*, p. 152. New York: McGraw-Hill Publishing Co., 1989.

Sokoloff, Leon. "Joint Diseases and Injuries," *Encyclopaedia Britannica Macropaedia*, v. 10, pp. 259-265. Chicago: Encyclopaedia Britannica, Inc. 1974.

Chapter Three

Gordon, Neil F. *Arthritis: Your Complete Exercise Guide*. Champaign, Illinois: Human Kinetics Publishers, 1993.

The Harvard Medical School Health Publications Group. *Arthritis: A Harvard Health Letter Special Report*. Boston: Harvard Medical School Health Publications Group, 1995.

The Harvard Medical School Health Publications Group. "Acupuncture," *Harvard Health Letter*, v. 18, no. 10 (Aug. 1993), pp. 6-8.

"Hydrotherapy," *Encyclopaedia Britannica Micropaedia*, v. V, p. 246.

Physicians' Desk Reference, 47th Edition. Montvale, N.J.: Medical Economics Data, 1993.

Schumacher, H. Ralph (ed.). *Primer on the Rheumatic Diseases, 10th Edition*. Atlanta: Arthritis Foundation, 1993.

Weinstein, Louis. "Antibiotic," *Encyclopaedia Britannica Macropaedia*, v.1, p. 986. Chicago: Encyclopaedia Britannica, Inc., 1974.

Chapter Four

Baigent, Margaret J. "Vitamin," *Encyclopaedia Britannica Macropaedia*, v. 19, pp. 488-493. Chicago: Encyclopaedia Britannica, Inc., 1974.

Barboriak, J. J. and Krehl, W. A. "Effect of Ascorbic Acid in Pantothenic Acid Deficiency," *Journal of Nutrition*, v. 63 (1957), pp. 601-609.

Bean, W. B. and Hodges, R. E. "Pantothenic Acid Deficiency Induced in Human Subjects," *Proceedings of the Society for Experimental Biology and Medicine*, v. 86 (1954), pp. 693-698.

Ershoff, B. H., Slater, R. B. A., and Gaines, J. G. "Effects of Pantothenic Acid Deficiency on Pituitary-Adrenal Function in the Rat," *Journal of Nutrition*, v. 50 (1953), pp. 299-316.

Fox, H. M. "Pantothenic Acid," *Handbook of Vitamins: Nutritional, Biochemical, and Clinical Aspects*, ed. Lawrence J. Machlin, ch. 11, pp. 437-457. New York: Marcel Dekker, Inc. 1984.

Fox, H. M. and Linkswiler, H. "Pantothenic Acid on Three Levels of Intake," *Journal of Nutrition*, v. 75 (1961), pp. 451-454.

Hodges, R. E., Ohlson, M. A., and Bean, W. B. "Pantothenic Acid Deficiency in Man," *Journal of Clinical Investigation*, v. 37 (1958), pp. 1642-1657.

Kutsky, R. J. *Handbook of Vitamins and Hormones*. New York: Van Nostrand Reinhold Co., 1973.

Marks, John. *A Guide to the Vitamins*, p. 6, pp. 126-130. Lancaster, England: Medical and Technical Publishing Co. Ltd., 1975.

Merck & Co., Inc. *Pantothenic Acid: Annotated Bibliography*. Rahway, N.J.: Merck & Co., Inc., February 1941.

Merck & Co. Inc. *Physiological Activity and Experimental Clinical Use of Calcium Pantothenate (Dextrorotatory)*. Rahway, N.J.: Merck & Co., Inc., March 1941.

Mills, R. C., Shaw, J. H., Elvehjem, C. A., and Phillips, P. H. "Curative Effects of Pantothenic Acid on Adrenal Necrosis," *Proceedings of the Society for Experimental Biology and Medicine*, v. 45 (1940), pp. 482-484.

Morgan, A. F. and Simms, H. D. "Adrenal Atrophy and Senescence Produced by a Vitamin Deficiency," *Science*, v. 89, no. 2320 (June 16, 1939), pp. 565-566.

Nelson, M. M., Sulon, E., Becks, H., Wainwright, W. W., and Evans, H. M. "Changes in Endochondral Ossification of the Tibia Accompanying Acute Pantothenic Acid Deficiency in Young Rats," *Proceedings of the Society for Experimental Biology and Medicine*, v. 73 (1950), pp. 31-36.

Novelli, G. D. "Metabolic Functions of Pantothenic Acid," *Physiological Review*, v. 33 (1953), pp. 525-543.

"Pantothenic Acid," *Encyclopaedia Britannica Micropaedia* v. VII, 726-727. Chicago: Encyclopaedia Britannica, Inc., 1974.

Pudelkewicz, C. and Roderuck, C. "Pantothenic Acid Deficiency in the Young Guinea Pig," *Journal of Nutrition*, v. 70 (1960) pp. 348-352.

Sheppard, A. J. and Johnson, B. C. "Pantothenic Acid Deficiency in the Growing Calf," *Journal of Nutrition*, v. 61 (1957), pp. 195-205.

Supplee, G. C., Bender, R. C., and Kahlenberg, O. J. "Interrelated Vitamin Requirements: Kidney Damage, Adrenal Hemorrhage and Cardiac Failure Correlated with Inadequacy of Pantothenic Acid," *Endocrinology*, v. 30, no. 3 (March, 1942), pp. 355-364.

Tarr, J. B., Tamura, T., and Stokstad, E. L. R. "Availability of Vitamin B_6 and Pantothenate in an Average American Diet in Man," *American Journal of Clinical Nutrition*, v. 34 (July, 1981), pp.1328-1337.

Vitamins in Medicine: Helsinki, 1985, ed. J. J. Himberg, W. Tackmann, D. Banks, pp. 9-10. Braunschweig/Wiesbaden, Germany: Friedrich Vieweg & Sohn, 1986.

Winters, R. H., Schultz, R. B., and Krehl, W. A. "The Adrenal Cortex of the Pantothenic Acid-Deficient Rat: Eosinophile and Lymphocyte Responses," *Endocrinology*, v. 50 (April, 1952), pp. 377-384.

Winters, R. H., Schultz, R. B., and Krehl, W. A. "The Adrenal Cortex of the Pantothenic Acid-Deficient Rat: Carbohydrate Metabolism," *Endocrinology*, v. 50 (April, 1952), pp. 388-398.

Chapter Five

"...and folic acid to prevent cleft palate," in "Nutrition," *Science News*, v. 148, no. 6 (Aug. 19, 1995), p. 127.

Barton-Wright, E.C. and Elliott, W.A. "The Pantothenic Acid Metabolism of Rheumatoid Arthritis," *The Lancet*, Oct. 26, 1963, pp. 862-863.

Carnation Nonfat Dry Milk label, 1995.

Davis, Donald B. Personal correspondence, 1995.

"Dietetics," *1946 Britannica Book of the Year*. Chicago: Encyclopedia Britannica, Inc., 1946, p. 264.

Eaton, S. Boyd and Konner, Melvin. "Paleolithic Nutrition: A Consideration of Its Nature and Current Implications," *The New England Journal of Medicine*, v. 312, no. 5 (Jan. 31, 1985), pp. 283-288.

"Dietary Supplements," *FDA Consumer*, Nov. 1993

Fox, Hazel Metz. "Pantothenic Acid," *Handbook of Vitamins: Nutritional, Biochemical, and Clinical Aspects*, edited by Lawrence J. Machlin. New York: Marcel Dekker, Inc., 1984. pp. 437-457.

Fox, Hazel Metz and Linkswiler, Hellen. "Pantothenic Acid Excretion on Three Levels of Intake," *Journal of Nutrition*, no. 75, 1961, pp. 451-454.

Hodges, R.E., Ohlson, M.A., and Bean, W. "Pantothenic Acid Deficiency in Man," *Journal of Clinical Investigation*, v. 37, 958, pp. 1642-1657.

Kalliomaki, J. L., Laine, V. A., and Markkanen, T. K. "Urinary Excretion of Thiamine, Riboflavin, Nicotinic Acid, and Pantothenic Acid in Patients with Rheumatoid Arthritis," *Acta Medica Scandinavica*, v. 166, fasc. 4, 1960.

Kutsky, Roman J. *Handbook of Vitamins and Hormones*. New York: Van Nostrand Reinhold, 1973.

Marks, John. *A Guide to the Vitamins*. Lancaster England: Medical and Technical Publishing Co. Ltd., 1975.

Merck & Co., Inc. *Physiological Activity and Experimental Clinical Use of Calcium Pantothenate (Dextrorotatory)*. Rahway, N.J.: Merck & Co., Inc., 1941.

National Research Council. *Recommended Dietary Allowances, 10th Edition*. Washington: National Academy Press, 1989.

Nourse, Alan E. *The Body*. New York: Time, Inc., 1964.

Novelli, G. David. "Metabolic Functions of Pantothenic Acid," *Physiological Review*, v. 33 (Oct. 1953), pp. 525-543.

Ovaltine Rich Chocolate label, 1996.

Schmidt, Vagn. "The Excretion of Pantothenic Acid in the Urine in Young and Old Individuals," *Journal of Gerontology*, v. 6 (1951), pp. 132-134.

Schroeder, Henry A. "Losses of Vitamins and Trace Minerals Resulting from Processing and Preservation of Food," *The American Journal of Clinical Nutrition*, v. 24 (May 1971), pp. 562-573.

Sebrell, William H. and Haggerty, James J. *Food and Nutrition*. New York: Time, Inc., 1967.

Sherlock, Sheila. "Liver, Human," *Encyclopaedia Britannica Macropaedia*, v. 10, p. 1224. Chicago: Encyclopaedia Britannica, Inc., 1974.

"Some Facts and Myths of Vitamins," *FDA Consumer*, Sept. 1979.

Srinivasan, V., Christensen, N., Wyse, B. W., and Hansen, R. G." Pantothenic Acid Nutritional Status in the Elderly—Institutionalized and Noninstitutionalized," *The American Journal of Clinical Nutrition*, v. 34 (Sept. 1981), pp. 1736-1742.

Supplee, G. C., Bender, R. C., and Kahlenberg, O. J. "Interrelated Vitamin Requirements: Kidney Damage, Adrenal Hemorrhage and Cardiac Failure Correlated with Inadequacy of Pantothenic Acid," *Endocrinology*, v. 30, no. 3 (March, 1942), pp. 355-364.

Tarr, J. B., Tamura, T., and Stokstad, E. L. R. "Availability of B_6 and Pantothenate in an Average American Diet in Man," *The American Journal of Clinical Nutrition*, v. 34 (July 1981), pp. 1328-1337.

University of California at Berkeley Wellness Letter. Vitamin Report. A report prepared by the editors of the *University of California at Berkeley Wellness Letter*. Berkeley: 1994.

Walsh, J. H., Wyse, B. W., and Hansen, R. G. "Pantothenic Acid Content of 75 Processed and Cooked Foods," *Journal of the American Dietetic Association*, v. 78 (Feb. 1981), pp. 140-144.

Williams, Roger J. *Nutrition Against Disease*. New York: Pitman Publishing Group, 1971.

Williams, Roger J. *Physician's Handbook of Nutritional Science*. Springfield, IL: Charles C. Thomas, 1975.

Williams, Roger J. *The Wonderful World Within You*. Wichita, KS: Bio-Communications Press, 1987.

Chapter Six

Annand, J.C. "Osteoarthrosis and Pantothenic Acid," *Journal of the College of General Practitioners*, v. 5 (1962), pp. 136-137.

Annand, J.C. "Pantothenic Acid and Osteoarthrosis" (Letter to the Editor), *The Lancet*, Nov. 30, 1963.

Aprahamian, Marc, et al. "Effects of Supplemental Pantothenic Acid on Wound Healing: Experimental Study in Rabbit," *The American Journal of Clinical Nutrition*, v. 41 (March 1985), pp. 578-589.

Barton-Wright, E.C. and Elliott, W.A. "The Pantothenic Acid Metabolism of Rheumatoid Arthritis," *The Lancet*, Oct. 26, 1963, pp. 862-863.

Barton-Wright, E.C., Elliot, W.A., and Reynolds E.B. Article in *Laboratory Practice*, v. 16 (1967), p. 699; reported in "Metabolic Treatment Corrects Arthritis Imbalance," *Medical World News*, Oct. 7, 1966, pp. 122-123.

Fox, Hazel Metz. "Pantothenic Acid," *Handbook of Vitamins: Nutritional, Biochemical, and Clinical Aspects*, edited by Lawrence J. Machlin. New York: Marcel Dekker, Inc., 1984. pp. 437-457.

Gardner, Thomas S. "The Use of Drosophila Melanogaster as a Screening Agent for Longevity Factors," *Journal of Gerontology*, v. 3, no. 1 (Jan. 1948), pp. 1-13.

General Practitioner Research Group. "Calcium Pantothenate in Arthritic Conditions," *Practitioner*, v. 224 (Feb. 1980), pp. 208-211.

Grenier, J. F., et al. "Pantothenic Acid (Vitamin B_5) Efficiency on Wound Healing," *Acta Vitaminologica et Enzymologica*, v. 4, no. 1-2 (1982), pp. 81-85

Haslock, D.I. and Wright, V. "Pantothenic Acid in the Treatment of Osteoarthrosis," *Rheumatology and Physical Medicine*, v. 11, (Feb. 1971), pp. 10-13.

Heiby, Walter A. *The Reverse Effect*. Deerfield, IL: Mediscience Publishers, 1988.

Hurley, L. S. and Morgan, A. F. "Carbohydrate Metabolism and Adrenal Cortical Function in the Pantothenic-Acid Deficient Rat," *Journal of Biological Chemistry*, v. 195 (1952), pp. 582-590.

Kalliomaki, J. L., Laine, V. A., and Markkanen, T. K. "Urinary Excretion of Thiamine, Riboflavin, Nicotinic Acid, and Pantothenic Acid in Patients with Rheumatoid Arthritis," *Acta Medica Scandinavica*, v. 166, fasc. 4, 1960.

Kutsky, R. J. *Handbook of Vitamins and Hormones*. New York: Van Nostrand Reinhold Co., 1973.

Marks, John. *A Guide to the Vitamins*, p. 6, pp. 126-130. Lancaster, England: Medical and Technical Publishing Co. Ltd., 1975.

Moiseenok, A.G. et al. "Anti-Inflammatory and Coenzyme Activity of Derivatives of Pantothenic Acid Under Conditions of Adjuvant Arthritis," *Pharmaceutical Chemistry Journal*, v. 15, no. 6 (1981), pp. 423-427.

Moiseenok, A. G. Personal correspondence, 1994.

Novelli, G. D. "Metabolic Functions of Pantothenic Acid," *Physiological Review*, v. 33 (1953), pp. 525-543.

Nelson, M. M., Sulon, E., Becks, H., Wainwright, W. W., and Evans, H. M. "Changes in Endochondral Ossification of the Tibia Accompanying Acute Pantothenic Acid Deficiency in Young Rats," *Proceedings of the Society for Experimental Biology and Medicine*, v. 73 (1950), pp. 31-36.

Otrokov, A. N. and Kopelevich, V. M. "On the Action of Pantothenic Acid on Inflammatory Process," *Chemistry, Biochemical Functions, and Application of Pantothenic Acid.* Minsk: Science and Engineering Publishers, Sept. 1977.

Ovesen, Lars. "Vitamin Therapy in the Absence of Obvious Deficiency: What Is the Evidence?" *Drugs,* v. 27 (1984), pp. 148-170.

Selye, Hans. "Effect of ACTH and Cortisone upon an Anaphylactoid Reaction," *The Canadian Medical Association Journal,* v. 61, no. 6 (Dec. 1949).

Szorady, I., Torvath, E., and Toth, E. "Uber die Antihistaminwirkung der Pantothensaure" ("On the Antihistamine Effect of Pantothenic Acid"), *International Journal for Vitamin Research,* v. 36 (1966), pp. 126-133.

University of California at Berkeley Wellness Letter. Vitamin Report. A report prepared by the editors of the *University of California at Berkeley Wellness Letter.* Berkeley: 1994.

Vaxman, F., et al. "Effect of Pantothenic Acid and Ascorbic Acid Supplementation on Human Skin Wound Healing," *European Surgical Research,* v. 27 (1995), pp. 158-166.

Welsh, Ashton L. "Lupus Erythematosus: Treatment by Combined Use of Massive Amounts of Pantothenic Acid and Vitamin E," *Archives of Dermatology,* v. 70 (1954), pp. 181-198.

Williams, Melvin H. "Vitamin Supplementation and Athletic Performance," *Elevated Dosages of Vitamins,* edited by Paul Walter, Hannes Stahelin, and Georg Brubacher. Lewiston, NY: Hans Huber Publishers, 1989.

Williams, R. J. and Pelton, R. B. "Effect of Pantothenic Acid on the Longevity of Mice," *Proceedings of the Society for Experimental Biology and Medicine,* v. 99 (1958), pp. 632-633.

Williams, Roger J. *Physician's Handbook of Nutritional Science.* Springfield, IL: Charles C. Thomas, 1975.

Williams, Roger J. *The Wonderful World Within You.* Wichita, KS: Bio-Communications Press, 1987.

Chapter Eight

Barton-Wright, E. C. and Elliott, W. A. "The Pantothenic Acid Metabolism of Rheumatoid Arthritis," *The Lancet*, Oct. 26, 1963, pp. 862-863.

Carnation Nonfat Dry Milk (label)

Davis, Donald B. Personal correspondence.

"Dietary Supplements," *FDA Consumer*, Nov. 1993

"Dietetics," *1946 Britannica Book of the Year*. Chicago: Encyclopaedia Britannica, Inc., 1946.

Eaton, S. Boyd and Konner, Melvin. "Paleolithic Nutrition: A Consideration of Its Nature and Current Implications," *The New England Journal of Medicine*, v. 312, no. 5 (Jan. 31, 1985), pp. 283-288.

Fox, H. M. "Pantothenic Acid," *Handbook of Vitamins: Nutritional, Biochemical, and Clinical Aspects*, ed. Lawrence J. Machlin. New York: Marcel Dekker, Inc. 1984, Chapter 11, pp. 437-457.

Heiby, Walter A. *The Reverse Effect*. Deerfield, IL: Mediscience Publishers, 1988.

Kutsky, R. J. *Handbook of Vitamins and Hormones*. New York: Van Nostrand Reinhold Co., 1973.

Marks, John. A *Guide to the Vitamins*. Lancaster, England: Medical and Technical Publishing Co. Ltd., 1975, p. 6, pp. 126-130.

Marks, John. "The Safety of Vitamins: an Overview," *Elevated Dosages of Vitamins*, edited by Paul Walter, Hannes Stahelin, and Georg Brubacher. Lewiston, NY: Hans Huber Publishers. 1989.

"Metabolic Treatment Corrects Arthritis Imbalance," *Medical World News*, Oct. 7, 1966, pp. 122-123.

Moiseenok, A.G. et al. "Anti-Inflammatory and Coenzyme Activity of Derivatives of Pantothenic Acid Under Conditions of Adjuvant Arthritis," *Pharmaceutical Chemistry Journal*, v. 15, no. 6 (1981), pp. 423-427.

Moiseenok, A. G. Personal correspondence, 1994.

National Research Council. *Recommended Dietary Allowances, 10th Edition*. Washington: National Academy Press, 1989

Otrokov, A. N. and Kopelevich, V. M. "On the Action of Pantothenic Acid on Inflammatory Process," *Chemistry, Biochemical Functions, and Application of Pantothenic Acid*. Minsk: Science and Engineering Publishers, Sept. 1977.

University of California at Berkeley Wellness Letter. Vitamin Report. A report prepared by the editors of the *University of California at Berkeley Wellness Letter*. Berkeley: 1994.

"Vitamin A Excess," *Encyclopaedia Britannica Micropaedia*, v. X, p. 467. Chicago: Encyclopaedia Britannica, Inc., 1974.

"Vitamin D Excess," *Encyclopaedia Britannica Micropaedia*, v. X, p. 470. Chicago: Encyclopaedia Britannica, Inc., 1974.

Welsh, Ashton L. "Lupus Erythematosus: Treatment by Combined Use of Massive Amounts of Pantothenic Acid and Vitamin E," *Archives of Dermatology* v. 70 (1954), pp. 181-198.

Williams, Melvin H. "Vitamin Supplementation and Athletic Performance," *Elevated Dosages of Vitamins*, edited by Paul Walter, Hannes Stahelin, and Georg Brubacher. Lewiston, NY: Hans Huber Publishers, 1989.

Williams, Roger J. *Physician's Handbook of Nutritional Science*. Springfield, IL: Charles C. Thomas, 1975.

Chapter Nine

Arthritis Foundation. *Arthritis: Unproven Remedies*. Atlanta: The Arthritis Foundation, 1987.

The Harvard Medical School Health Publications Group. *Arthritis: A Harvard Health Letter Special Report*. Boston: Harvard Medical School Health Publications Group, 1995.

Panush, Richard M., MD. "Nontraditional Remedies," *Primer on the Rheumatic Diseases, Tenth Edition*, ed. H. Ralph Schumacher. Atlanta: The Arthritis Foundation, 1993.

Welsh, Ashton L. "Lupus Erythematosus: Treatment by Combined Use of Massive Amounts of Pantothenic Acid and Vitamin E," *Archives of Dermatology*, v. 70 (1954), pp. 181-198.

Chapter Ten

Jones, Gail J., Secretary to the Membership Administration Manager, Royal Society of Chemistry. Personal correspondence, Aug. 10, 1995.

Beckwith, Julie, Assistant Librarian, Royal College of Physicians. Personal correspondence, July 21, 1995.

Williams, Roger J. *Physician's Handbook of Nutritional Science*. Springfield, IL: Charles C. Thomas Publisher, 1975.

Appendix

Annand, J. C. "Osteoarthrosis and Pantothenic Acid," *Journal of the College of General Practitioners*, v. 5 (1962), pp. 136-137.

Barton-Wright, E. C. and Elliott, W. A. "The Pantothenic Acid Metabolism of Rheumatoid Arthritis," *The Lancet*, Oct. 26, 1963, pp. 862-863.

Brandt, K. D. and Slemenda, C. W. "Osteoarthritis: A. Epidemiology, Pathology, and Pathogenesis." *Primer on the Rheumatic Diseases, Tenth Edition*, ed. H. Ralph Schumacher. Atlanta: The Arthritis Foundation, 1993.

General Practitioners Research Group. "Calcium Pantothenate in Arthritis Conditions," *Practitioner*, v. 224 (Feb. 1980), pp. 208-211.

Kalliomaki, J. L., Laine, V. A., and Markkanen, T. K. "Urinary Excretion of Thiamine, Riboflavin, Nicotinic Acid, and Pantothenic Acid in Patients with Rheumatoid Arthritis," *Acta Medica Scandinavica*, v. 166, fasc. 4, 1960.

Moiseenok, A. G. et al. "Anti-Inflammatory and Coenzyme Activity of Derivatives of Pantothenic Acid Under Conditions of Adjuvant Arthritis," *Pharmaceutical Chemistry Journal*, v. 15, no. 6 (1981), pp. 423-427.

Wilder, R. L. "Rheumatoid Arthritis: A. Epidemiology, Pathology, and Pathogenesis," *Primer on the Rheumatic Diseases, Tenth Edition*, ed. H. Ralph Schumacher. Atlanta: The Arthritis Foundation, 1993.

INDEX